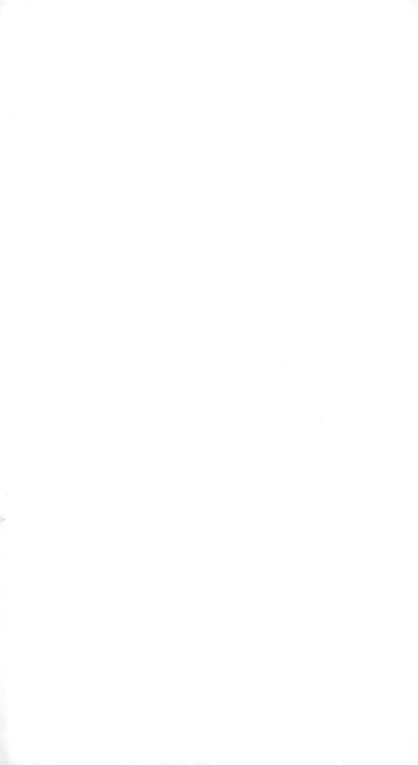

Anatomy in Your Pocket

Edited by
Anne M. Gilroy, MA
Professor
Department of Radiology
University of Massachusetts Medical School
Worcester, Massachusetts

Based on the work of
Michael Schuenke, MD, PhD
Institute of Anatomy
Christian Albrecht University Kiel
Kiel, Germany

Erik Schulte, MD
Department of Functional and Clinical Anatomy
University Medicine
Johannes Gutenberg University
Mainz, Germany

Udo Schumacher, MD, FRCPath, CBiol, FSB, DSc
Institute of Anatomy and Experimental Morphology
Center for Experimental Medicine
University Cancer Center
University Medical Center Hamburg-Eppendorf
Hamburg, Germany

Illustrations by
Markus Voll
Karl Wesker

442 illustrations

Thieme
New York • Stuttgart • Delhi • Rio de Janeiro

Executive Editor: Delia DeTurris
Managing Editor: Torsten Scheihagen
Director, Editorial Services: Mary Jo Casey
Production Editor: Barbara Chernow
International Production Director: Andreas Schabert
Editorial Director: Sue Hodgson
International Marketing Director: Fiona Henderson
International Sales Director: Louisa Turrell
Director of Institutional Sales: Adam Bernacki
Senior Vice President and Chief Operating Officer:
    Sarah Vanderbilt
President: Brian D. Scanlan

Library of Congress Cataloging-in-Publication Data

Names: Gilroy, Anne M., editor. | Voll, Markus M.,
    illustrator. | Wesker, Karl, illustrator. | Based
    on (work): Schuenke, Michael. Thieme atlas of
    anatomy.
Title: Anatomy in your pocket / edited by Anne M.
    Gilroy ; based on the work of Michael
    Schuenke, Erik Schulte, Udo Schumacher ;
    illustrations by Markus Voll, Karl Wesker.
Description: New York : Thieme, [2018] |
Identifiers: LCCN 2017056187 (print) | LCCN
    2017057413 (ebook) | ISBN 9781626239135
    () | ISBN 9781626239128 (alk. paper) | ISBN
    9781626239135 (ebook)
Subjects: | MESH: Anatomy | Handbooks | Atlases
Classification: LCC QM25 (ebook) | LCC QM25
    (print) | NLM QS 39 | DDC 612.0022/3—dc23
LC record available at https://lccn.loc.gov/
    2017056187

Copyright © 2018 by Thieme Medical Publishers, Inc.

Thieme Publishers New York
333 Seventh Avenue, New York, NY 10001 USA
+1 800 782 3488, customerservice@thieme.com

Thieme Publishers Stuttgart
Rüdigerstrasse 14, 70469 Stuttgart, Germany
+49 [0]711 8931 421, customerservice@thieme.de

Thieme Publishers Delhi
A-12, Second Floor, Sector-2, Noida-201301
Uttar Pradesh, India
+91 120 45 566 00, customerservice@thieme.in

Thieme Publishers Rio de Janeiro, Thieme
Publicações Ltda.
Edifício Rodolpho de Paoli, 25º andar
Av. Nilo Peçanha, 50 – Sala 2508,
Rio de Janeiro 20020-906 Brasil
+55 21 3172-2297 / +55 21 3172-1896

Cover design: Thieme Publishing Group
Typesetting by Carol Pierson, Chernow Editorial
    Services, Inc.

Printed in India by Replika Press Pvt. Ltd.   5 4 3 2 1

ISBN 978-1-62623-912-8

Also available as an e-book:
eISBN 978-1-62623-913-5

Important note: Medicine is an ever-changing science undergoing continual development. Research and clinical experience are continually expanding our knowledge, in particular our knowledge of proper treatment and drug therapy. Insofar as this book mentions any dosage or application, readers may rest assured that the authors, editors, and publishers have made every effort to ensure that such references are in accordance with **the state of knowledge at the time of production of the book.**

Nevertheless, this does not involve, imply, or express any guarantee or responsibility on the part of the publishers in respect to any dosage instructions and forms of applications stated in the book. **Every user is requested to examine carefully** the manufacturers' leaflets accompanying each drug and to check, if necessary in consultation with a physician or specialist, whether the dosage schedules mentioned therein or the contraindications stated by the manufacturers differ from the statements made in the present book. Such examination is particularly important with drugs that are either rarely used or have been newly released on the market. Every dosage schedule or every form of application used is entirely at the user's own risk and responsibility. The authors and publishers request every user to report to the publishers any discrepancies or inaccuracies noticed. If errors in this work are found after publication, errata will be posted at www.thieme.com on the product description page.

Some of the product names, patents, and registered designs referred to in this book are in fact registered trademarks or proprietary names even though specific reference to this fact is not always made in the text. Therefore, the appearance of a name without designation as proprietary is not to be construed as a representation by the publisher that it is in the public domain.

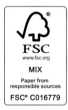

"It is not length of life,
but depth of life that matters."
                    ~Ralph Waldo Emerson

To Luke, thank you for the inspiration of a life lived
with courage and grace,

And

To Laila, Harvey, Eva, and Finn, the future is yours.

Contents

Icon Key

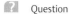 Question

Answer

Comment

Clinical

Each card in this set features a full-color illustration with key structures labeled numerically. The reverse side of every card lists the labels. Where questions appear on the front of the card, corresponding answers are supplied on the back. Comments provide helpful information, and clinical correlates describe relevant applications of anatomy.

Back

Bony Vertebral Column

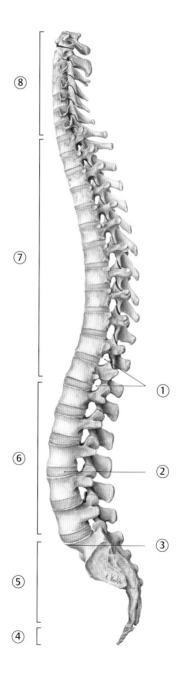

Bony Vertebral Column

① intervertebral foramina

② intervertebral disc

③ sacral promontory

④ coccyx

⑤ sacrum (S1–S5 vertebrae)

⑥ L1–L5 vertebrae

⑦ T1–T12 vertebrae

⑧ C1–C7 vertebrae

❄ The characteristic curvatures of the adult spine appear over the course of postnatal development, being only partially present in a newborn. The newborn has a kyphotic spinal curvature; lumbar lordosis develops later and becomes stable at puberty.

Fig. 2.1B. From *Atlas of Anatomy, Third Edition*, p. 4.

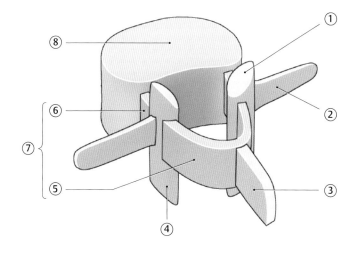

Structural Elements of a Vertebra

① superior articular process

② transverse process

③ spinous process

④ inferior articular process

⑤ lamina

⑥ pedicle

⑦ vertebral arch

⑧ vertebral body

�֎ With the exception of the atlas (C1) and axis (C2), all vertebrae consist of the same structural elements. The pedicles and laminae make up the vertebral arch, which, together with the vertebral body, encloses the vertebral foramen. The combined vertebral foramina of all of the vertebrae create the vertebral canal.

Fig. 2.4. From *Atlas of Anatomy, Third Edition*, p. 7.

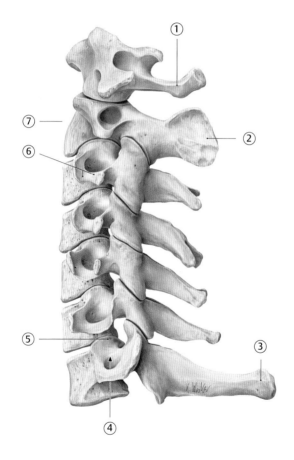

Cervical Spine

1.   posterior arch of atlas
2.   spinous process of C2
3.   spinous process of C7
4.   transverse foramen
5.   uncinate process
6.   groove for spinal n.
7.   C2 (axis)

The cervical spine is prone to hyperextension injuries, such as whiplash, which can occur when the head extends back much farther than it normally would. The most common injuries of the cervical spine are fractures of the dens of the atlas, traumatic spondylolisthesis (anterior slippage of a vertebral body), and atlas fractures. Patient prognosis largely depends on the spinal level of the injury.

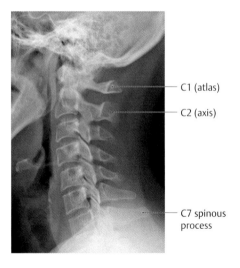

C1 (atlas)

C2 (axis)

C7 spinous process

Fig. 2.6A,B. From *Atlas of Anatomy, Third Edition*, p. 8.

Atlas

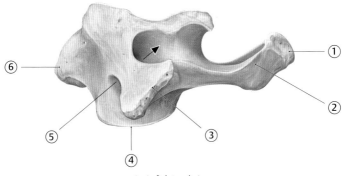

A. Left lateral view

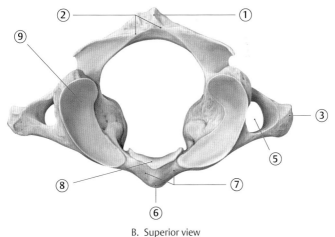

B. Superior view

How does the basic structure of the atlas (C1) differ from typical cervical vertebrae?

Atlas

① posterior tubercle
② posterior arch
③ transverse process
④ inferior articular facet
⑤ transverse foramen
⑥ anterior tubercle
⑦ anterior arch
⑧ facet for den
⑨ superior articular facet

The atlas lacks a vertebral body and a spinous process characteristic of C2–C7. Superiorly it articulates with the occipital condyles of the occipital bone of the skull.

Axis

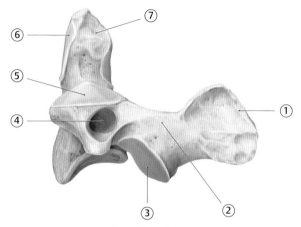

A. Left lateral view

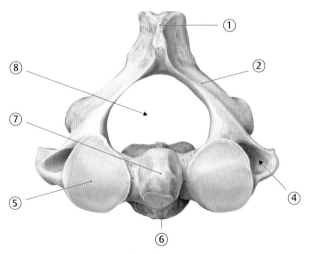

B. Superior view

Axis

①   spinous process

②   vertebral arch

③   inferior articular facet

④   transverse foramen

⑤   superior articular facet

⑥   anterior articular facet

⑦   dens

⑧   vertebral foramen

The axis is unique among vertebrae in having a superiorly projecting process, the dens, which articulates with the anterior arch of the atlas.

Typical Cervical Vertebra (C4)

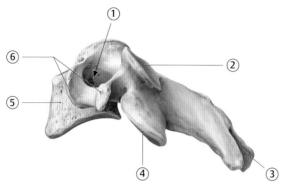

A. Left lateral view

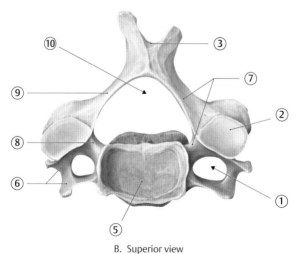

B. Superior view

What structure is transmitted through the transverse foramina of most (usually C1–C6) cervical vertebrae?

Typical Cervical Vertebra (C4)

① transverse foramen

② superior articular facet

③ spinous process

④ inferior articular facet

⑤ body

⑥ transverse process

⑦ vertebral arch

⑧ pedicle

⑨ lamina

⑩ vertebral foramen

❗ The vertebral arteries, which originate from the subclavian arteries, pass through the transverse foramina of C1–C6.

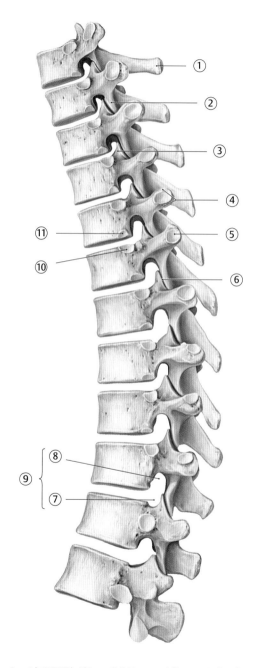

Thoracic Spine

1. spinous process
2. inferior articular process
3. superior articular process
4. transverse process
5. costal facet on transverse process
6. zygapophyseal joint
7. superior vertebral notch
8. inferior vertebral notch
9. intervertebral foramen
10. superior costal facet
11. inferior costal facet

Fig. 2.10. From *Atlas of Anatomy, Third Edition*, p. 10.

Lumbar Spine

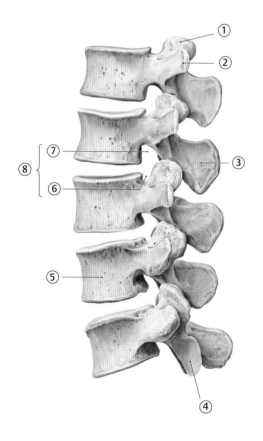

Lumbar Spine

① superior articular process
② transverse process
③ spinous process
④ inferior articular facet
⑤ vertebral body
⑥ superior vertebral notch
⑦ inferior vertebral notch
⑧ intervertebral foramen

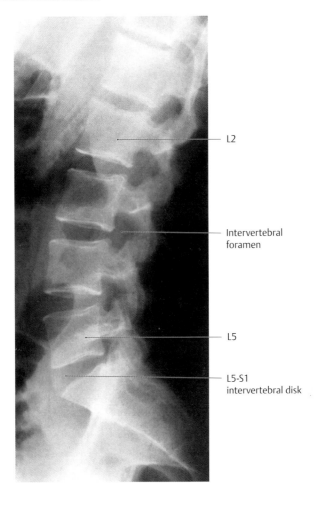

L2

Intervertebral
foramen

L5

L5-S1
intervertebral disk

Fig. 2.12 and Clinical Box 2.3A. From *Atlas of Anatomy, Third Edition*, p. 11.

Sacrum and Coccyx, Anterior View

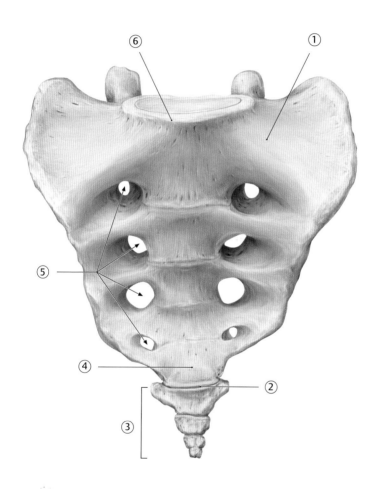

What structures pass through the anterior sacral foramina?

Sacrum and Coccyx, Anterior View

① wing of sacrum

② sacrococcygeal joint

③ coccyx

④ apex of sacrum

⑤ anterior sacral foramina

⑥ promontory

⚠ Anterior rami of the sacral spinal nerves pass through the anterior foramina to join the sacral plexus.

Fig. 2.14A. From *Atlas of Anatomy, Third Edition*, p. 12.

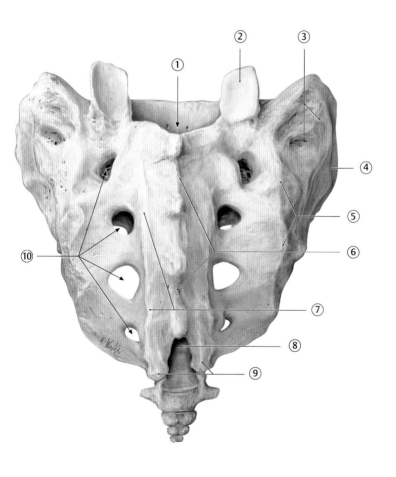

Sacrum and Coccyx, Posterior View

Fig. 2.14B. From *Atlas of Anatomy, Third Edition*, p. 12.

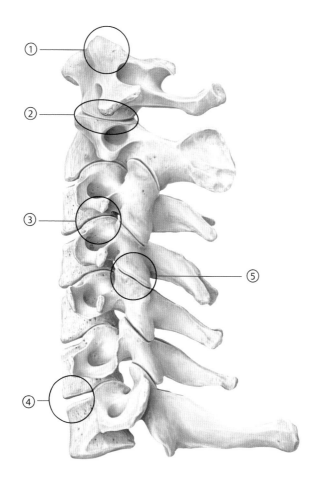

Joints of the Vertebral Column

①   atlantooccipital joint

②   atlantoaxial joint

③   uncovertebral joint

④   intervertebral joint

⑤   zygopophyseal joint

Craniovertebral joints	
Atlanto-occipital joints	Occiput–C1
Atlantoaxial joints	C1–C2
Joints of the vertebral bodies	
Uncovertebral joints	C3–C7
Intervertebral joints	C2–S1
Joints of the vertebral arch	
Zygapophyseal joints	C2–S1

Table 2.2. From *Atlas of Anatomy, Third Edition*, p. 16.

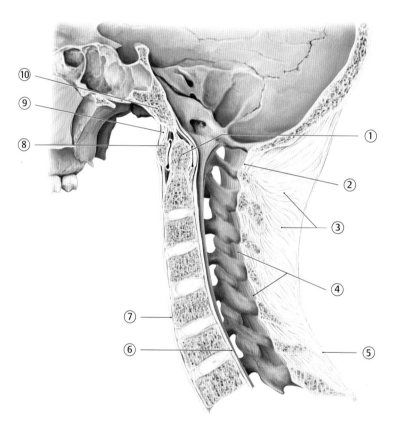

Ligaments of the Cervical Spine

① dens of axis (C2)

② posterior atlanto-occipital membrane

③ nuchal lig.

④ ligamenta flava

⑤ supraspinous lig.

⑥ posterior longitudinal lig.

⑦ anterior longitudinal lig.

⑧ anterior arch of atlas (C1)

⑨ anterior atlanto-occipital membrane

⑩ occipital bone

The nuchal ligament is the broadened, sagittally oriented part of the supraspinous ligament that extends from the vertebra prominens (C7) to the external occipital protuberance.

Fig. 2.28A. From *Atlas of Anatomy, Third Edition*, p. 21.

Ligaments of the Vertebral Column: Thoracolumbar Junction

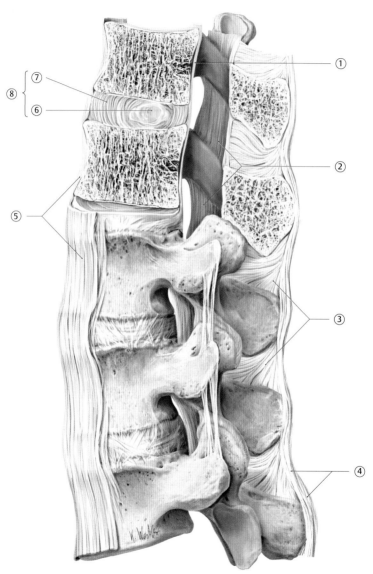

Left lateral view T11–T13; midsagittal section T11–T12

Ligaments of the Vertebral Column: Thoracolumbar Junction

① posterior longitudinal lig.

② ligamenta flava

③ interspinous ligs.

④ supraspinous lig.

⑤ anterior longitudinal lig.

⑥ nucleus pulposus

⑦ anulus fibrosus

⑧ intervertebral disk

❋ The ligaments of the spinal column bind the vertebrae securely to one another and enable the spine to withstand high mechanical loads and shearing stresses.

Fig. 2.29. From *Atlas of Anatomy, Third Edition*, p. 22.

Short Nuchal and Craniovertebral Joint Muscles

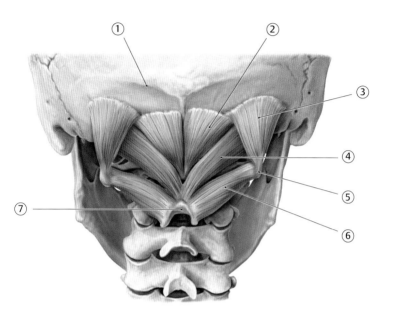

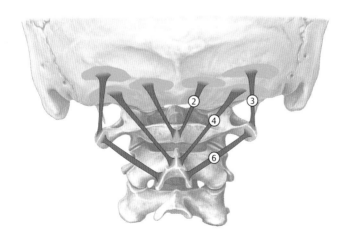

Short Nuchal and Craniovertebral Joint Muscles

①   superior nuchal line

②   rectus capitis posterior minor

③   obliquus capitis superior

④   rectus capitis posterior major

⑤   transverse process of atlas (C1)

⑥   obliquus capitis inferior

⑦   spinous process of axis (C2)

Muscle		Origin	Insertion	Innervation	Action
Rectus capitis posterior	Rectus capitis posterior major	C2 (spinous process)	Occipital bone (inferior nuchal line, middle third)		*Bilateral:* Extends head *Unilateral:* Rotates head to same side
	Rectus capitis posterior minor	C1 (posterior tubercle)	Occipital bone (inferior nuchal line, inner third)		
Obliquus capitis	Obliquus capitis superior	C1 (transverse process)	Occipital bone (inferior nuchal line, middle third; above rectus capitis posterior major)	C1 (posterior ramus = suboccipital n.)	*Bilateral:* Extends head *Unilateral:* Tilts head to same side; rotates to opposite side
	Obliquus capitis inferior	C2 (spinous process)	C1 (transverse process)		*Bilateral:* Extends head *Unilateral:* Rotates head to same side

Superficial Intrinsic Back Muscles

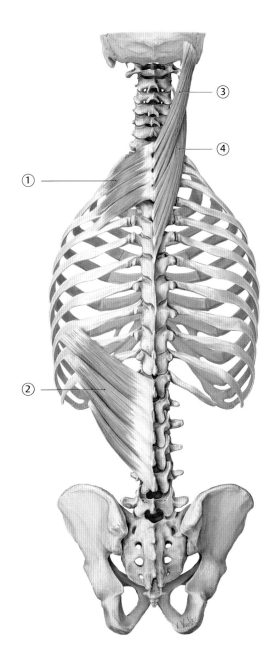

Superficial Intrinsic Back Muscles

①   serratus posterior superior

②   serratus posterior inferior

③   splenius capitis

④   splenius cervicis

Muscle		Origin	Insertion	Innervation	Action
Serratus posterior	Serratus posterior superior	Nuchal lig.; C7–T3 (spinous processes)	2nd–4th ribs (superior borders)	Spinal nn. T2–T5 (anterior rami)	Elevates ribs
	Serratus posterior inferior	T11–L2 (spinous processes)	8th–12th ribs (inferior borders, near angles)	Spinal nn. T9–T12 (anterior rami)	Depresses ribs
Splenius	Splenius capitis	Nuchal lig.; C7–T3 or T4 (spinous processes)	Lateral third nuchal line (occipital bone); mastoid process (temporal bone)	Spinal nn. C1–C6 (posterior rami, lateral branches)	*Bilateral:* Extends cervical spine and head *Unilateral:* Flexes and rotates head to the same side
	Splenius cervicis	T3–T6 or T7 (spinous processes)	C1–C3/4 (transverse processes)		

Fig. 3.10A. From *Atlas of Anatomy, Third Edition,* p. 33.

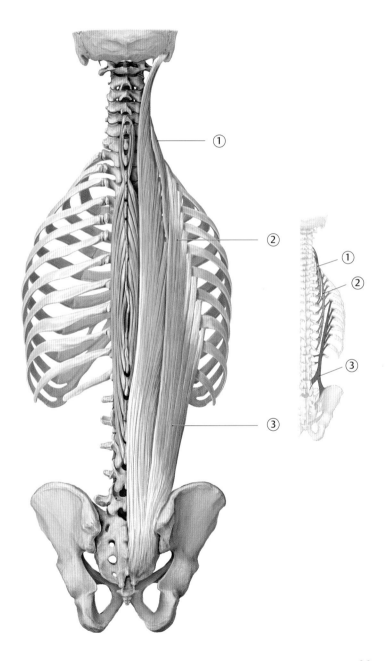

Intermediate Intrinsic Back Muscles I

①   iliocostalis cervicis

②   iliocostalis thoracis

③   iliocostalis lumborum

Muscle		Origin	Insertion	Innervation	Action
Iliocostalis	① Iliocostalis cervicis	3rd–7th ribs	C4–C6 (transverse processes)	Spinal nn. C8–L1 (posterior rami, lateral branches)	*Bilateral:* Extends spine *Unilateral:* Bends spine laterally to same side
	② Iliocostalis thoracis	7th–12th ribs	1st–6th ribs		
	③ Iliocostalis lumborum	Sacrum; iliac crest; thoracolumbar fascia (posterior layer)	6th–12th ribs; thoracolumbar fascia (posterior layer); upper lumbar vertebrae (transverse processes)		

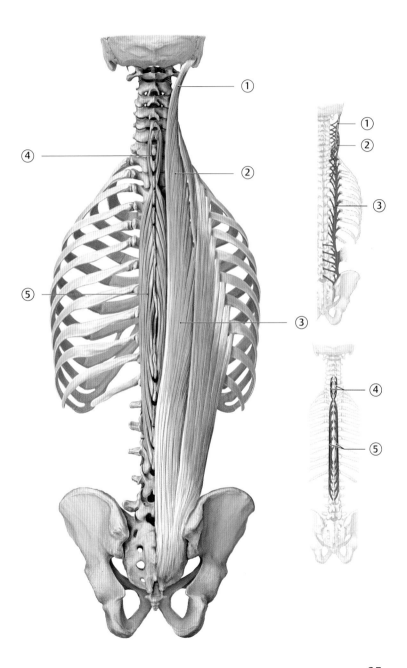

Intermediate Intrinsic Back Muscles II

① longissimus capitis
② longissimus cervicis
③ longissimus thoracis
④ spinalis cervicis
⑤ spinalis thoracis

Muscle		Origin	Insertion	Innervation	Action
Longissimus	Longissimus capitis	T1–T3 (transverse processes); C4–C7 (transverse and articular processes)	Temporal bone (mastoid process)	Spinal nn. C1–L5 (posterior rami, lateral branches)	*Bilateral:* Extends head *Unilateral:* Flexes and rotates head to same side
	Longissimus cervicis	T1–T6 (transverse processes)	C2–C5 (transverse processes)		*Bilateral:* Extends spine *Unilateral:* Bends spine laterally to same side
	Longissimus thoracis	Sacrum; iliac crest; lumbar vertebrae (spinous processes); lower thoracic vertebrae (transverse processes)	2nd–12th ribs; thoracic and lumbar vertebrae (transverse processes)		
Spinalis	Spinalis cervicis	C5–T2 (spinous processes)	C2–C5 (spinous processes)	Spinal nn. (posterior rami)	*Bilateral:* Extends cervical and thoracic spine *Unilateral:* Bends cervical and thoracic spine to same side
	Spinalis thoracis	T10–L3 (spinous processes, lateral surfaces)	T2–T8 (spinous processes, lateral surfaces)		

Fig. 3.9B,C, 3.10B. From *Atlas of Anatomy, Third Edition*, p. 32–33.

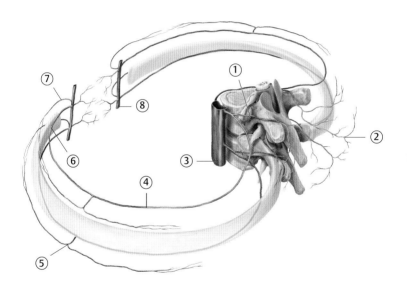

Posterior Intercostal Arteries

①   dorsal branch of posterior intercostal a.

②   medial cutaneous branch

③   thoracic aorta

④   posterior intercostal a.

⑤   lateral cutaneous branch

⑥   anterior intercostal a.

⑦   anterior cutaneous branch

⑧   internal thoracic a.

❄ The structures of the back are supplied by branches of the posterior intercostal arteries, which arise from the thoracic aorta or the subclavian artery. They give rise to cutaneous and muscular branches as well as spinal branches, which supply the spinal cord.

Fig. 4.1C. From *Atlas of Anatomy, Third Edition*, p. 36.

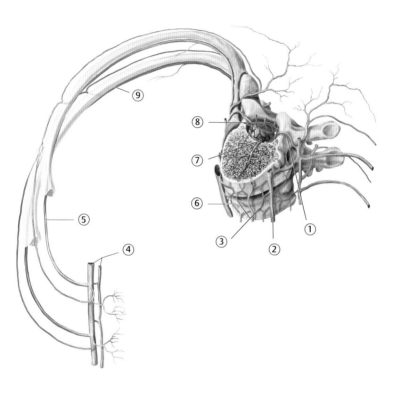

Posterior Intercostal Veins

① intervertebral v.
② hemiazygos v.
③ anterior external vertebral venous plexus
④ internal thoracic vv.
⑤ anterior intercostal v.
⑥ azygos v.
⑦ anterior external vertebral venous plexus
⑧ posterior internal vertebral venous plexus
⑨ posterior intercostal v.

✳ The veins of the back drain into the azygos vein via the superior intercostal veins, hemiazygos veins, and ascending lumbar veins. The interior of the spinal column is drained by the vertebral venous plexus, which runs the length of the spine.

Fig. 4.2C. From *Atlas of Anatomy, Third Edition*, p. 37.

Spinal Meningeal Layers

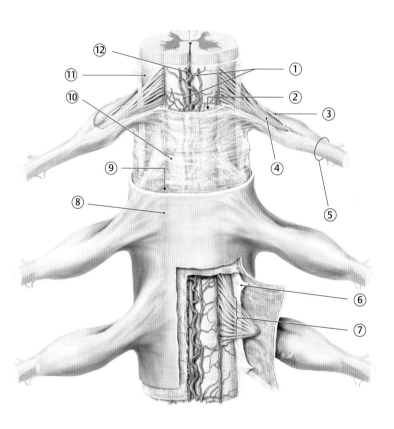

Spinal Meningeal Layers

① anterior spinal vv.
② subarachnoid space
③ posterior root
④ anterior root
⑤ spinal n.
⑥ denticulate lig.
⑦ anterior rootlets
⑧ dura mater
⑨ subdural space
⑩ arachnoid (mater)
⑪ pia mater
⑫ anterior spinal a.

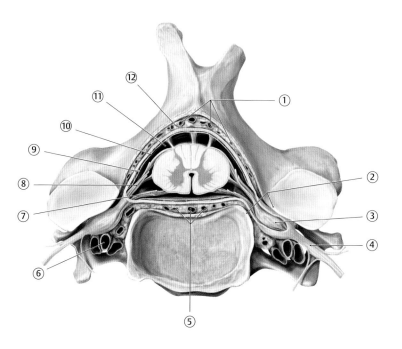

What is contained in the epidural and subarachnoid spaces surrounding the spinal cord?

Cervical Spinal Cord In Situ: Transverse Section

①   posterior internal vertebral venous plexus

②   intervertebral foramen

③   spinal ganglion

④   spinal n.

⑤   anterior internal vertebral venous plexus

⑥   vertebral a.

⑦   anterior root

⑧   posterior root

⑨   dura mater

⑩   arachnoid (mater)

⑪   subarachnoid space

⑫   epidural space

! The epidural space contains fat and the internal vertebral venous plexus. The subarachnoid space contains the cerebrospinal fluid and is traversed by the denticulate ligaments, which anchor the pia mater to the dura.

Fig. 4.8. From *Atlas of Anatomy, Third Edition*, p. 40.

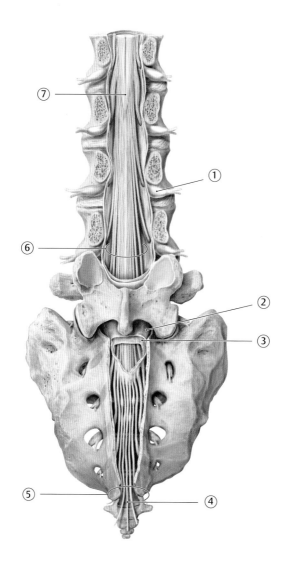

Cauda Equina in the Vertebral Canal

1. spinal ganglion
2. dura mater
3. arachnoid (mater)
4. filum terminale
5. sacral hiatus
6. cauda equina
7. conus medullaris

⚕ Although the spinal cord ends at the conus medullaris, the lower spinal roots, L2–Co1 (known as the cauda equina), extend inferiorly within the lumbar cistern, an expansion of the subarachnoid space surrounded by the dural sac.

Fig. 4.9. From *Atlas of Anatomy, Third Edition*, p. 41.

Spinal Cord Segment

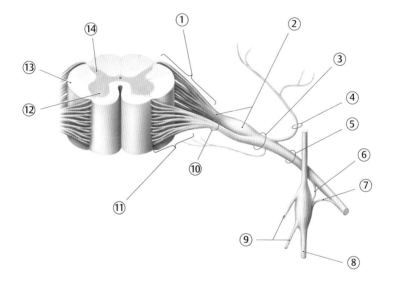

🖼 What is the destination of the anterior and posterior rami of the spinal nerves?

Spinal Cord Segment

①   posterior rootlets

②   posterior root with spinal ganglion

③   spinal n.

④   posterior ramus

⑤   anterior ramus

⑥   gray ramus communicans

⑦   white ramus communicans

⑧   sympathetic trunk

⑨   splanchnic nn.

⑩   anterior root

⑪   anterior rootlets

⑫   gray matter, anterior horn

⑬   white matter

⑭   gray matter, posterior horn

Anterior rami innervate the anterolateral trunk wall and limbs:
- C1–C4 form the cervical plexus
- C5–T1 form the brachial plexus
- T1–T12 remain as segmental (intercostal) nn.
- L1–L4 become the lumbar plexus
- L5–S3 become the sacral plexus

Posterior rami innervate the skin and muscles of the back and posterior scalp.

Fig. 4.12. From *Atlas of Anatomy, Third Edition*, p. 42.

Thorax

(Continued)

Thorax

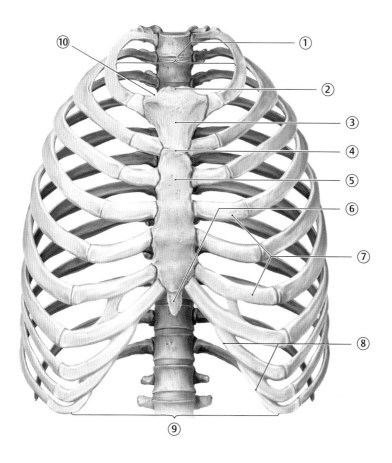

Distinguish between true, false, and floating ribs.

Thoracic Skeleton

① superior thoracic aperture
② jugular notch
③ manubrium
④ sternal angle
⑤ body
⑥ xiphoid process
⑦ costal cartilage
⑧ costal margin (arch)
⑨ inferior thoracic aperture
⑩ clavicular notch

🛇 True ribs (1–7) attach to the sternum via individual costal cartilages. False ribs (8–10) attach to the sternum indirectly though costal cartilages that connect to the one superior to it. Floating ribs (11–12) have no costal cartilage and are not connected to the sternum.

Fig. 7.1. From *Atlas of Anatomy, Third Edition*, p. 56.

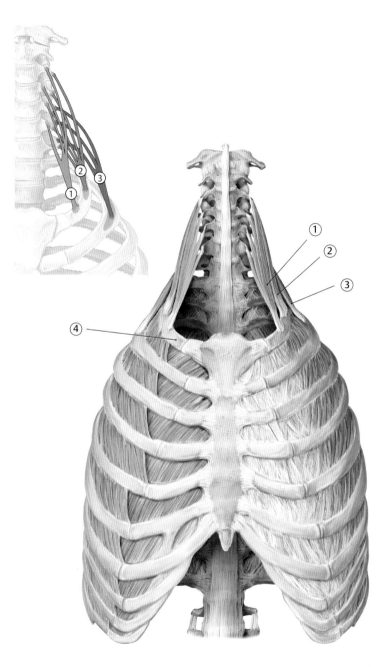

Muscles of the Thoracic Wall I

①   anterior scalene

②   middle scalene

③   posterior scalene

④   1st rib

Muscle		Origin	Insertion	Innervation	Action
Scalene mm.	Anterior scalene m.	C3–C6 (transverse processes, anterior tubercles)	1st rib (anterior scalene tubercle)	Anterior rami of C4–C6 spinal nn.	*With ribs mobile:* Raises upper ribs (inspiration) *With ribs fixed:* Bends cervical spine to same side (unilateral); flexes neck (bilateral)
	Middle scalene m.	C3–C7 (transverse processes, posterior tubercles)	1st rib (posterior to groove for subclavian a.)	Anterior rami of C3–C8 spinal nn.	
	Posterior scalene m.	C5–C7 (transverse processes, posterior tubercles)	2nd rib (anterior scalene tubercle)	Anterior rami of C6 or C7–C8 spinal nn.	

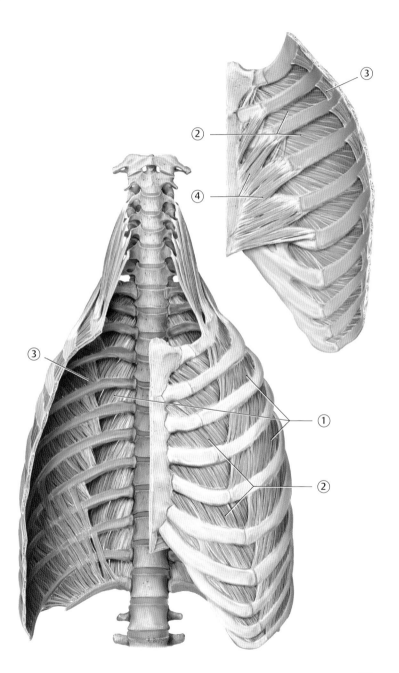

Muscles of the Thoracic Wall II

① external intercostal mm.

② internal intercostal mm.

③ innermost intercostal mm.

④ transversus thoracis

Muscle		Origin	Insertion	Innervation	Action
Intercostal mm.	External intercostal mm.	Lower margin of rib to upper margin of next lower rib (courses obliquely forward and downward from costal tubercle to chondro-osseous junction)		1st–11th intercostal nn.	Raises ribs (inspiration); supports intercostal spaces; stabilizes chest wall
	Internal intercostal mm.	Lower margin of rib to upper margin of next lower rib (courses obliquely forward and upward from costal angle to sternum			Lowers ribs (expiration); supports intercostal spaces; stabilizes chest wall
	Innermost intercostal mm.				
Subcostal mm.		Lower margin of lower ribs to inner surface of ribs two to three ribs below		Adjacent intercostal nn.	Lowers ribs (expiration)
Transversus thoracis m.		Sternum and xiphoid process (inner surface)	2nd–6th ribs (costal cartilage, inner surface)	2nd–6th intercostal nn.	Weakly lowers ribs (expiration)

Fig. 7.11. From *Atlas of Anatomy, Third Edition*, p. 63.

Diaphragm, Coronal Section

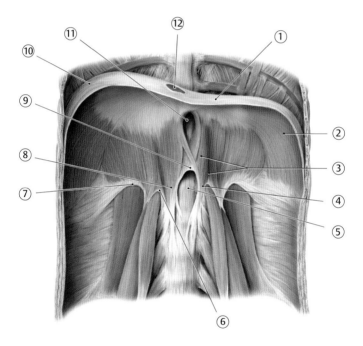

Diaphragm, Coronal Section

① central tendon

② costal part

③ lumbar part

④ left crus

⑤ aortic hiatus

⑥ medial arcuate lig.

⑦ lateral arcuate lig.

⑧ right crus

⑨ median arcuate lig.

⑩ right dome

⑪ esophageal hiatus

⑫ caval opening

Muscle		Origin	Insertion	Innervation	Action
Diaphragm	Costal part	7th–12th ribs (inner surface; lower margin of costal arch)	Central tendon	Phrenic n. (C3–C5, cervical plexus)	Principal muscle of respiration (diaphragmatic and thoracic breathing); aids in compressing abdominal viscera (abdominal press)
	Lumbar part	Medial part: L1–L3 vertebral bodies, intervertebral disks, and anterior longitudinal lig. as right and left crura			
		Lateral parts: lateral and medial arcuate ligs.			
	Sternal part	Xiphoid process (posterior surface)			

Fig. 7.12C. From *Atlas of Anatomy, Third Edition*, p. 64.

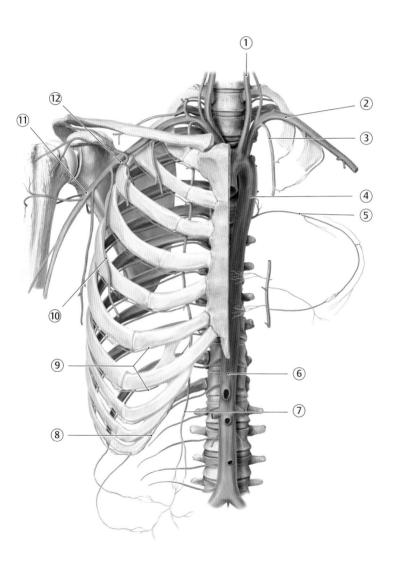

Arteries of the Thoracic Wall

①   left common carotid a.

②   left subclavian a.

③   internal thoracic a.

④   thoracic aorta

⑤   posterior intercostal a.

⑥   abdominal aorta

⑦   superior epigastric a.

⑧   musculophrenic a.

⑨   anterior intercostal a.

⑩   lateral thoracic a.

⑪   axillary a.

⑫   thoracoacromial a.

Origin	Branch
Axillary a.	Lateral thoracic a.
	Thoracoacromial a.
Subclavian a.	Posterior intercostal aa. (1st and 2nd)
	Superior thoracic a.
Thoracic aorta	Posterior intercostal aa. (3rd–12th)
Internal thoracic a.	Anterior intercostal aa.
	Musculophrenic a.
	Superior epigastric a.

Fig. 7.17. From *Atlas of Anatomy, Third Edition*, p. 68.

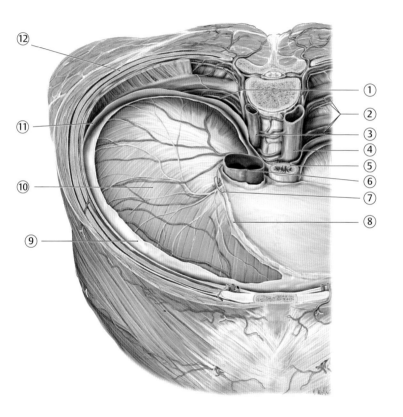

What nerve innervates the diaphragm, and from which spinal cord levels does it arise?

Neurovasculature of the Diaphragm

① intercostal nn.

② posterior intercostal aa. and vv.

③ azygos v.

④ thoracic aorta

⑤ esophagus

⑥ inferior vena cava

⑦ phrenic n., pericardiacophrenic a. and v.

⑧ pericardial sac

⑨ parietal pleura, diaphragmatic part

⑩ diaphragm

⑪ parietal pleura, costal part

⑫ external intercostal m.

❗ The phrenic nerve, which arises from the anterior rami of C3–C5, provides all of the motor and most of the sensory innervation to the diaphragm. Subcostal and lower intercostal nerves provide sensory innervation to the periphery of the diaphragm.

Fig. 7.27. From *Atlas of Anatomy, Third Edition*, p. 73.

Structures of the Breast

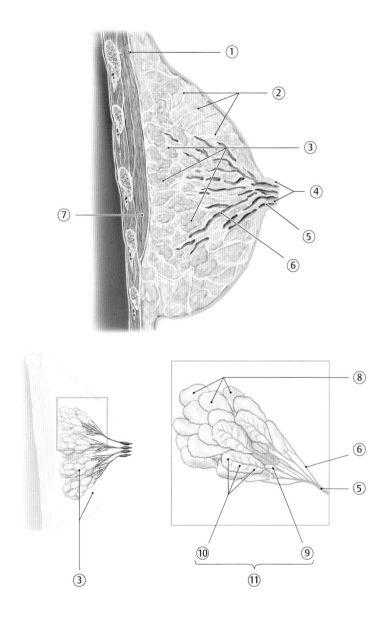

The lymphatic vessels of the breast drain primarily to which group of nodes?

Structures of the Breast

1. pectoral fascia
2. suspensory (Cooper) ligs.
3. mammary lobes
4. nipple
5. lactiferous sinus
6. lactiferous duct
7. pectoralis major
8. lobules
9. terminal duct
10. acini
11. terminal duct lobular unit (TDLU)

⚠️ Most lymph (75%) from the breast (particularly from the lateral quadrant) drains to axillary nodes. Lymph from the medial breast can drain to parasternal nodes and the contralateral breast. Some lymph may drain to deep pectoral or abdominal nodes.

The Aortic Arch

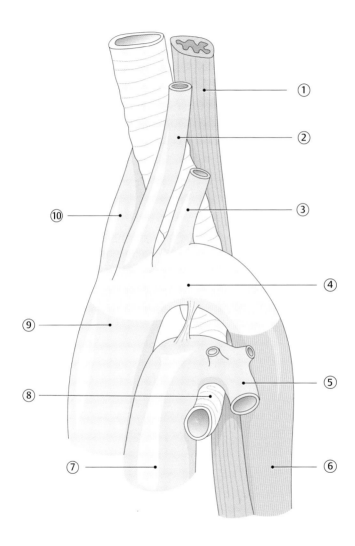

①

②

③

④

⑤

⑥

⑦

⑧

⑨

⑩

What skeletal landmark corresponds with the beginning and end of the aortic arch?

The Aortic Arch

① esophagus
② left common carotid a.
③ left subclavian a.
④ aortic arch
⑤ left pulmonary a.
⑥ descending aorta
⑦ pulmonary trunk
⑧ left main bronchus
⑨ ascending aorta
⑩ brachiocephalic trunk

❗ The sternal angle at vertebral level T4/T5 corresponds to the transition between the ascending aorta and aortic arch anteriorly, and the aortic arch and descending (thoracic) aorta posteriorly.

Fig. 8.4B. From *Atlas of Anatomy, Third Edition*, p. 81.

Azygos System

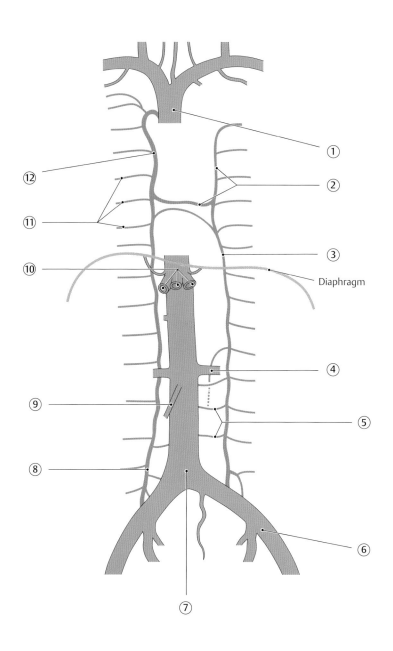

(1)

(2)

(3)

Diaphragm

(4)

(5)

(6)

(7)

(8)

(9)

(10)

(11)

(12)

Azygos System

① superior vena cava

② accessory hemiazygos v.

③ hemiazygos v.

④ left renal v.

⑤ lumbar vv.

⑥ left common iliac v.

⑦ inferior vena cava

⑧ right ascending lumbar v.

⑨ right gonadal v.

⑩ hepatic vv.

⑪ posterior intercostal vv.

⑫ azygos v.

❋ The azygos system forms an anastomosis between venous drainage of the head, neck, and upper limb (via the superior vena cava) and the drainage of the retroperitoneum of the abdomen and lower limbs (via the inferior vena cava).

Fig. 8.6. From *Atlas of Anatomy, Third Edition*, p. 83.

Lymphatic Trunks in the Thorax

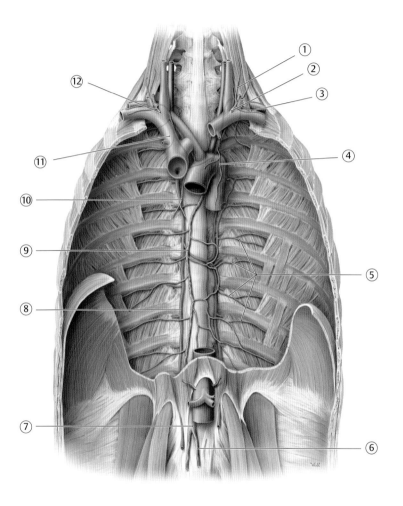

Which regions of the body are drained by the thoracic (left lymphatic) duct?

Lymphatic Trunks in the Thorax

①   jugular trunk

②   termination of the thoracic duct

③   subclavian trunk

④   left bronchomediastinal trunk

⑤   intercostal lymphatics

⑥   left lumbar trunk

⑦   cisterna chyli

⑧   azygos v.

⑨   thoracic duct

⑩   right bronchomediastinal trunk

⑪   right brachiocephalic v.

⑫   right lymphatic duct

! The body's chief lymphatic vessel, the thoracic duct, begins in the abdomen at the cisterna chyli. It drains lymph from all of the body below the diaphragm as well as the left side of the head, neck, and thorax. The remaining areas drain to the right lymphatic duct.

Fig. 8.7. From *Atlas of Anatomy, Third Edition*, p. 84.

Contents of the Mediastinum

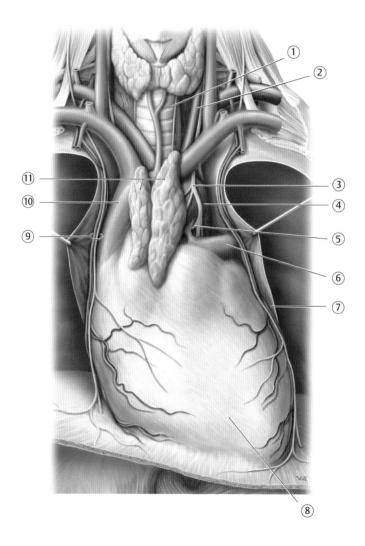

How is the mediastinum divided, and in which region is the heart located?

Contents of the Mediastinum

① trachea

② left common carotid a.

③ left vagus n.

④ aorta

⑤ left recurrent laryngeal n.

⑥ left pulmonary a.

⑦ parietal pleura, mediastinal part

⑧ fibrous pericardium

⑨ pericardiacophrenic a. and v., phrenic n.

⑩ superior vena cava

⑪ thymus

! The mediastinum is divided into superior and inferior regions by a horizontal plane at the T4/T5 level. The inferior mediastinum is further divided into anterior, middle and posterior parts. The heart, pericardium and great vessels are the primary structures within the middle mediastinum.

Fig. 9.2A. From *Atlas of Anatomy, Third Edition*, p. 89.

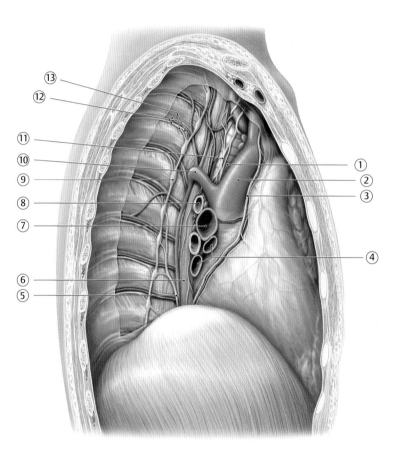

Mediastinum, Right Lateral View

① trachea

② superior vena cava

③ phrenic n.

④ right pulmonary vv.

⑤ greater splanchnic n.

⑥ esophagus

⑦ right pulmonary a.

⑧ superior lobar bronchus

⑨ sympathetic trunk, thoracic ganglion

⑩ azygos v.

⑪ right vagus n.

⑫ intercostal v., a., n.

⑬ white and gray rami communicans

Fig. 9.3A. From *Atlas of Anatomy, Third Edition*, p. 90.

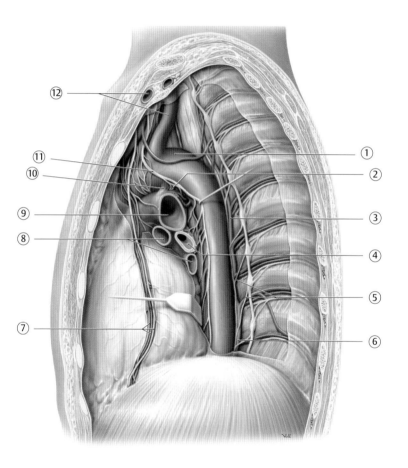

Mediastinum, Left Lateral View

1. aortic arch
2. left recurrent laryngeal n.
3. accessory hemiazygos v.
4. left main bronchus
5. splanchnic nn.
6. hemiazygos v.
7. phrenic n., pericardiacophrenic a. and v.
8. left pulmonary v.
9. left pulmonary a.
10. ligamentum arteriosum
11. left vagus n.
12. left subclavian a. and v.

Fig. 9.3B. From *Atlas of Anatomy, Third Edition*, p. 91.

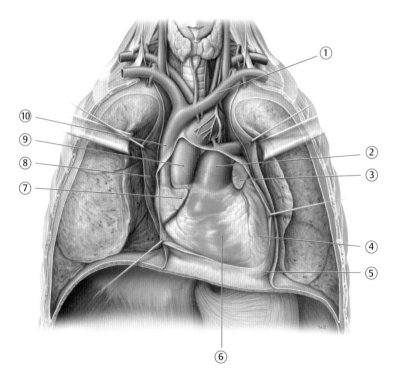

Describe the position of the heart relative to the thoracic skeleton.

Heart In Situ

1. left brachiocephalic v.
2. pulmonary trunk
3. left auricle
4. left ventricle
5. cardiac apex
6. right ventricle
7. right auricle
8. parietal pleura, mediastinal part
9. ascending aorta
10. superior vena cava

! The heart lies behind the sternum between the 2nd and 6th costal cartilages. It is located within the middle mediastinum and projects into the left side of the thoracic cavity. The apex lies approximately at the 5th left intercostal space.

Fig. 9.6B. From *Atlas of Anatomy, Third Edition*, p. 93.

Posterior Pericardium

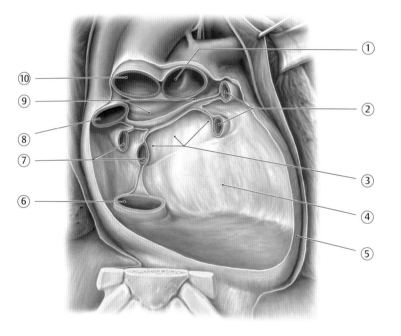

What is the transverse pericardial sinus?

Posterior Pericardium

1. pulmonary trunk
2. left pulmonary vv.
3. oblique pericardial sinus
4. serous pericardium, parietal layer
5. fibrous pericardium
6. inferior vena cava
7. right pulmonary vv.
8. superior vena cava
9. transverse pericardial sinus
10. ascending aorta

⚠️ The transverse pericardial sinus is the space that separates the heart's inflow tracts (superior vena cava and pulmonary veins) from its outflow tracts (aorta and pulmonary trunk).

Fig. 9.8. From *Atlas of Anatomy, Third Edition*, p. 94.

Anterior Surface of the Heart

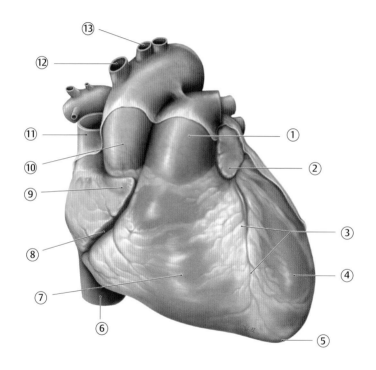

Which chamber(s) of the heart form(s) its sternocostal surface?

Anterior Surface of the Heart

① pulmonary trunk

② left auricle

③ anterior interventricular sulcus

④ left ventricle

⑤ cardiac apex

⑥ inferior vena cava

⑦ right ventricle

⑧ coronary (right atrioventricular) sulcus

⑨ right auricle

⑩ ascending aorta

⑪ superior vena cava

⑫ brachiocephalic trunk

⑬ left common carotid a.

! The sternocostal, or anterior, surface is formed primarily by the right ventricle with portions of the right atrium and left ventricle.

Fig. 9.11A. From *Atlas of Anatomy, Third Edition*, p. 96.

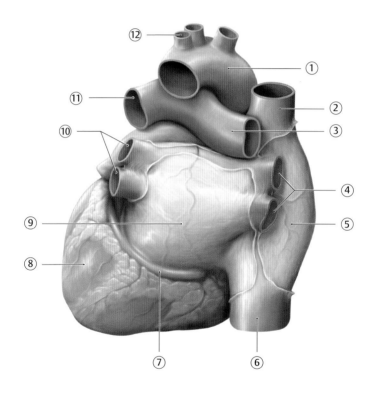

Which chambers of the heart form its diaphragmatic surface?

Posterior Surface (Base) of the Heart

①   aortic arch

②   superior vena cava

③   right pulmonary a.

④   right pulmonary vv.

⑤   right atrium

⑥   inferior vena cava

⑦   coronary sinus

⑧   left ventricle

⑨   left atrium

⑩   left pulmonary vv.

⑪   left pulmonary a.

⑫   left subclavian a.

❗ The right and left ventricles form the diaphragmatic surface of the heart.

Fig. 9.11B. From *Atlas of Anatomy, Third Edition*, p. 96.

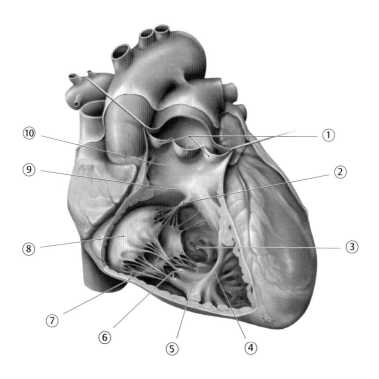

Right Ventricle of the Heart, Anterior View

1. valve of pulmonary trunk, cusps
2. septal papillary m.
3. interventricular septum
4. septomarginal trabecula (moderator band)
5. posterior papillary m.
6. anterior papillary m.
7. tendinous cords
8. right atrioventricular valve, anterior cusp
9. supraventricular crest
10. conus arteriosus (infundibulum)

Fig. 9.12A. From *Atlas of Anatomy, Third Edition*, p. 97.

Right Atrium of the Heart, Right Lateral View

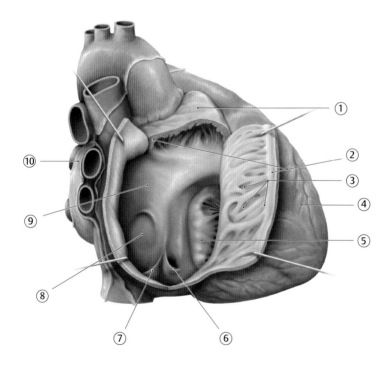

🔲 Which structure in the right atrium remains as a remnant of the embryonic communication between the right and left atria?

Right Atrium of the Heart, Right Lateral View

① right auricle

② terminal crest

③ pectinate mm.

④ right ventricle

⑤ right atrioventricular orifice with atrioventricular valve

⑥ valve of coronary sinus

⑦ valve of inferior vena cava

⑧ fossa ovalis (oval fossa)

⑨ interatrial septum

⑩ left atrium

⚠ The fossa ovalis, a depression in the atrial wall, is the remnant of the foramen ovale of the embryonic heart.

Fig. 9.12B. From *Atlas of Anatomy, Third Edition*, p. 97.

Left Atrium and Ventricle of the Heart, Left Lateral View

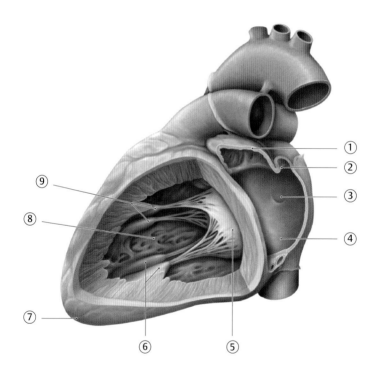

What is the function of the tendinous cords that attach to the cusps of the atrioventricular valves?

Left Atrium and Ventricle of the Heart, Left Lateral View

①   left auricle

②   left superior pulmonary v.

③   valve of fossa ovalis (oval fossa)

④   interatrial septum

⑤   left atrioventricular valve, cusp

⑥   posterior papillary m.

⑦   cardiac apex

⑧   trabeculae carneae of interventricular septum

⑨   anterior papillary m.

⚠ The tendinous cords attach the free edge of the valve leaflets to the papillary muscles. During contraction of the ventricles, they maintain closure of the valves, thus preventing regurgitation of blood back into the atria.

Fig. 9.12C. From *Atlas of Anatomy, Third Edition*, p. 97.

Cardiac Valves

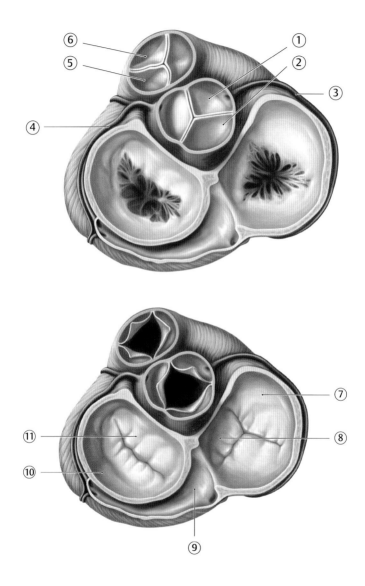

🔲 During which part of the cardiac cycle are the pulmonary and aortic valves closed (top image)?

Cardiac Valves

1. right cusp of aortic valve
2. posterior cusp of aortic valve
3. right coronary a.
4. left coronary a.
5. left cusp of pulmonary valve
6. anterior cusp of pulmonary valve
7. anterior cusp of right atrioventricular valve
8. septal cusp of right atrioventricular valve
9. coronary sinus
10. posterior cusp of left atrioventricular valve
11. anterior cusp of left atrioventricular valve

! The pulmonary and aortic valves are closed during diastole (relation of the ventricles).

Coronary Arteries and Cardiac Veins, Anterior View

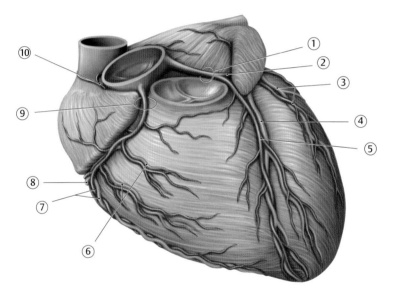

Which regions of the heart are supplied by the anterior interventricular artery?

Coronary Arteries and Cardiac Veins, Anterior View

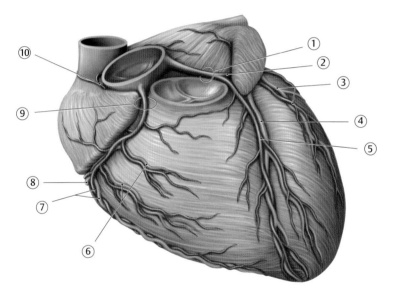

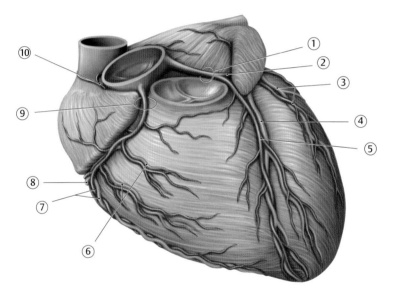

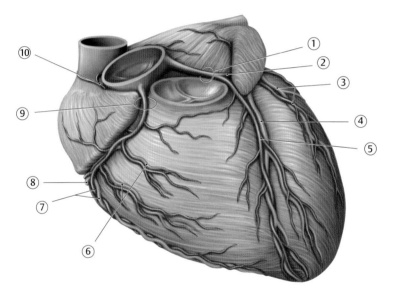

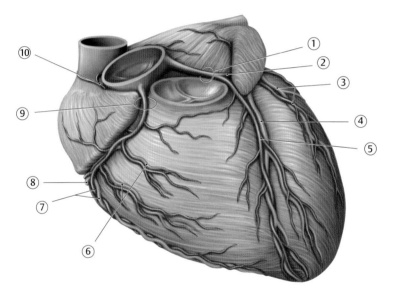

① left coronary a.

② circumflex branch

③ left marginal a. and v.

④ great cardiac v.

⑤ anterior interventricular branch (left anterior descending)

⑥ anterior vv. of right ventricle

⑦ right marginal a. and v.

⑧ small cardiac v.

⑨ right coronary a.

⑩ branch to sinoatrial node

⚠️ The anterior interventricular artery (left anterior descending; LAD), which arises from the left coronary artery, supplies the anterior walls of both ventricles and the anterior two thirds of the interventricular septum, including the atrioventricular (AV) bundles, which run within the septum.

Fig. 9.16A. From *Atlas of Anatomy, Third Edition*, p. 100.

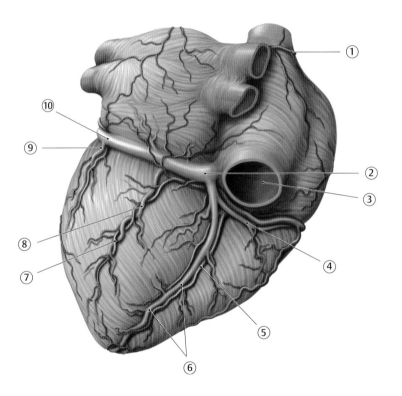

Where does the coronary sinus terminate?

Coronary Arteries and Cardiac Veins, Posteroinferior View

① branch to sinoatrial node

② coronary sinus

③ right coronary a.

④ small cardiac v.

⑤ posterior interventricular a. (posterior descending)

⑥ middle cardiac v.

⑦ right posterolateral a.

⑧ left posterior ventricular v.

⑨ left marginal v.

⑩ great cardiac v.

! The coronary sinus receives most of the venous drainage of the heart. It runs in the posterior coronary sulcus and terminates in the right atrium, where its orifice is guarded by the thebesian valve.

Fig. 9.16B. From *Atlas of Anatomy, Third Edition*, p. 100.

Cardiac Conduction System

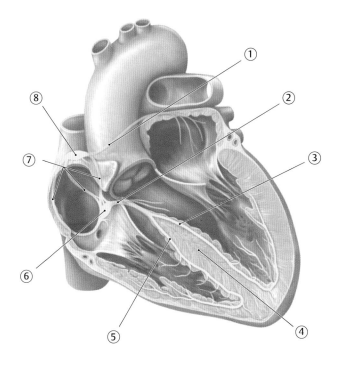

Why is the sinoatrial (SA) node known as the pacemaker of the heart?

Cardiac Conduction System

① interatrial bundle

② atrioventricular (AV) bundle (of His)

③ left bundle branch

④ interventricular septum

⑤ right bundle branch

⑥ atrioventricular (AV) node

⑦ anterior, middle, and posterior intermodal bundles

⑧ sinoatrial (SA) node

❗ The conduction system of the heart, innervated by the autonomic nerves of the cardiac plexus, generates and transmits impulses that modulate the contraction of the cardiac muscle. The sinoatrial (SA) node is known as the pacemaker of the heart because it initiates and transmits the impulses to the atria and atrioventricular (AV) node.

Fig. 9.18A. From *Atlas of Anatomy, Third Edition*, p. 102.

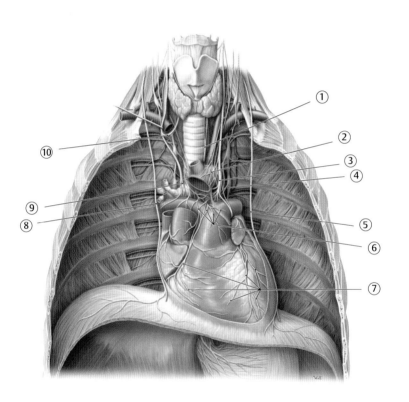

Autonomic Nerves of the Heart

① left recurrent laryngeal n.
② thoracic aortic plexus
③ left vagus n.
④ sympathetic trunk
⑤ left phrenic n.
⑥ pulmonary plexus
⑦ cardiac plexus
⑧ right phrenic n.
⑨ right vagus n.
⑩ right recurrent laryngeal n.

The heart receives sympathetic innervation via three cervical cardiac nerves as well as thoracic cardiac branches arising from T1–T6. Parasympathetic innervation arises from cervical and thoracic cardiac nerves, which arise from the vagus nerves. Both sympathetic and parasympathetic fibers contribute to the cardiac, aortic, and pulmonary plexuses.

Fig. 9.19C. From *Atlas of Anatomy, Third Edition*, p. 103.

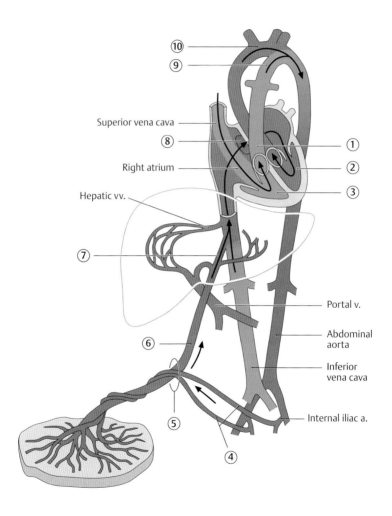

Superior vena cava

Right atrium

Hepatic vv.

Portal v.

Abdominal aorta

Inferior vena cava

Internal iliac a.

Prenatal Circulation

① pulmonary trunk
② left ventricle
③ right ventricle
④ umbilical aa.
⑤ umbilicus
⑥ umbilical v.
⑦ ductus venosus
⑧ oval foramen (open)
⑨ ductus arteriosus (patent)
⑩ aortic arch

Derivatives of fetal circulatory structures	
Fetal structure	**Adult remnant**
Ductus arteriosus	Ligamentum arteriosum
Foramen ovale	Fossa ovalis (oval fossa)
Ductus venosus	Ligamentum venosum
Umbilical v.	Round lig. of the liver (ligamentum teres)
Umbilical a.	Medial umbilical lig.

Fig. 9.20. From *Atlas of Anatomy, Third Edition*, p. 104.

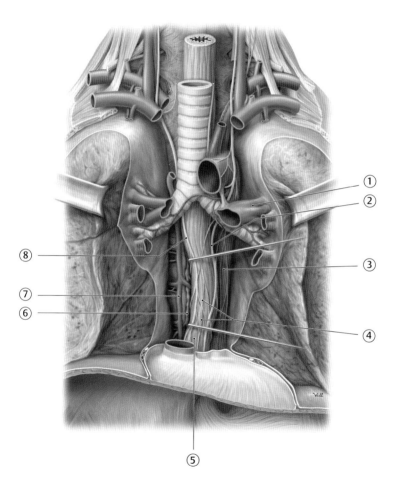

Esophagus In Situ

① left pulmonary a.

② left vagus n.

③ thoracic aorta

④ esophageal plexus

⑤ esophagus, thoracic part

⑥ thoracic duct

⑦ azygos v.

⑧ right vagus n.

The esophageal plexus is formed by the right and left vagus nerves (parasympathetic fibers) with contributions from the greater splanchnic nerve (sympathetic fibers).

Fig. 9.23. From *Atlas of Anatomy, Third Edition*, p. 106.

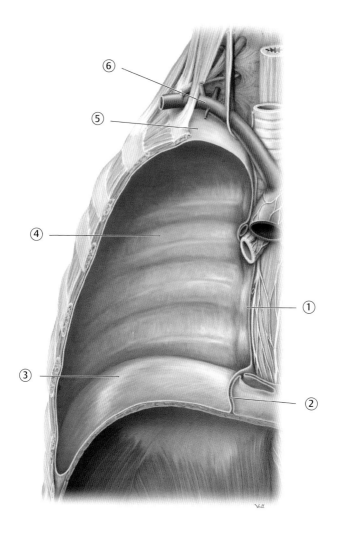

Parietal Pleura

1. mediastinal part
2. fibrous pericardium
3. diaphragmatic part
4. costal part
5. cervical part
6. subclavian a.

Fig. 10.2. From *Atlas of Anatomy, Third Edition*, p. 113.

Pleura and the Costodiaphragmatic Recess, Coronal Section, Anterior View

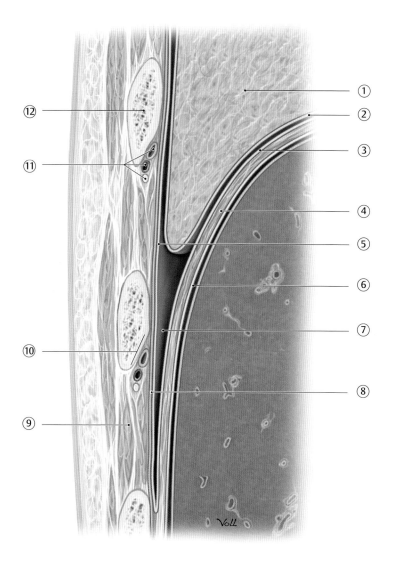

〘1〙

① ① ② ③ ④ ⑤ ⑥ ⑦ ⑧

⑫ ⑪ ⑩ ⑨

Pleura and the Costodiaphragmatic Recess, Coronal Section, Anterior View

1. right lung
2. visceral pleura
3. parietal pleura, diaphragmatic part
4. diaphragm
5. parietal pleura, costal part
6. peritoneum, diaphragmatic part
7. costodiaphragmatic recess
8. endothoracic fascia
9. external intercostal m.
10. costal groove
11. intercostal v., a., and n.
12. 8th rib

Fig. 7.24. From *Atlas of Anatomy, Third Edition*, p. 71.

Right Lung

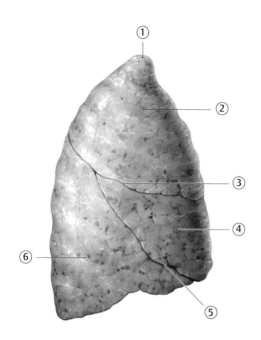

A. Lateral view

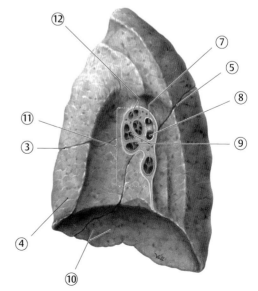

B. Medial view

Illustrator: Markus Voll

Right Lung

1. apex
2. superior lobe
3. horizontal fissure
4. middle lobe
5. oblique fissure
6. inferior lobe
7. superior lobar bronchus
8. inferior and middle lobar bronchi (common origin)
9. branches of right pulmonary vv.
10. diaphragmatic surface (base of lung)
11. hilum
12. branches of right pulmonary a.

Left Lung

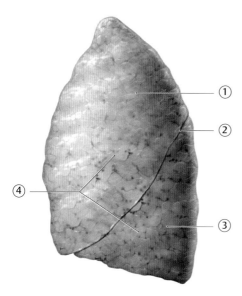

A. Lateral view

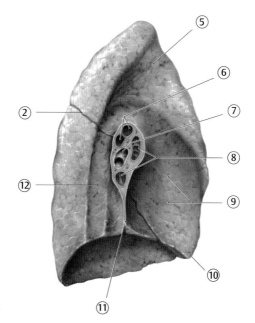

B. Medial view

Left Lung

① superior lobe
② oblique fissure
③ inferior lobe
④ costal surface
⑤ mediastinal surface
⑥ branches of left pulmonary a.
⑦ superior and inferior lobar bronchi
⑧ branches of left pulmonary v.
⑨ cardiac impression
⑩ lingula
⑪ pulmonary lig.
⑫ aortic impression

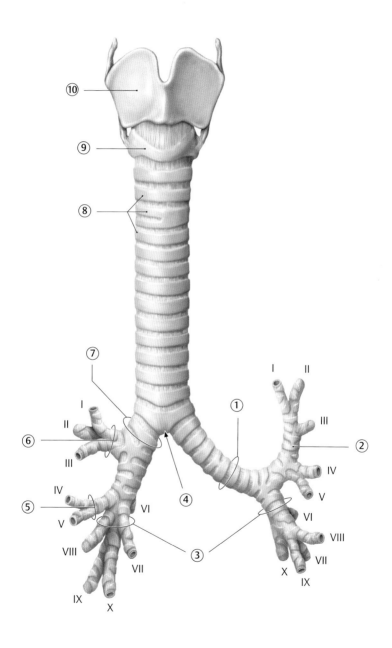

Trachea

1. left main bronchus
2. left superior lobar bronchus
3. right/left inferior lobar bronchi
4. tracheal bifurcation
5. right middle lobar bronchus
6. right superior lobar bronchus
7. right main bronchus
8. tracheal cartilages
9. cricoid cartilage
10. thyroid cartilage

Fig. 10.12B. From *Atlas of Anatomy, Third Edition*, p. 120.

Bronchial Tree: Conduction Portion

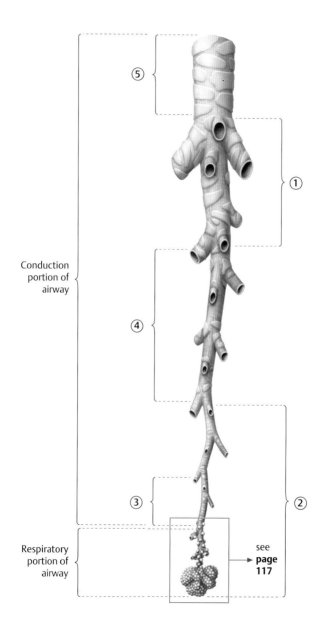

⑤

①

Conduction
portion of
airway

④

③

②

Respiratory
portion of
airway

see
► **page**
117

115

Bronchial Tree: Conduction Portion

①   large subsegmental bronchus
②   bronchiole
③   terminal bronchiole
④   small subsegmental bronchus
⑤   segmental bronchus

Fig. 10.13A. From *Atlas of Anatomy, Third Edition*, p. 121.

Bronchial Tree: Respiratory Portion

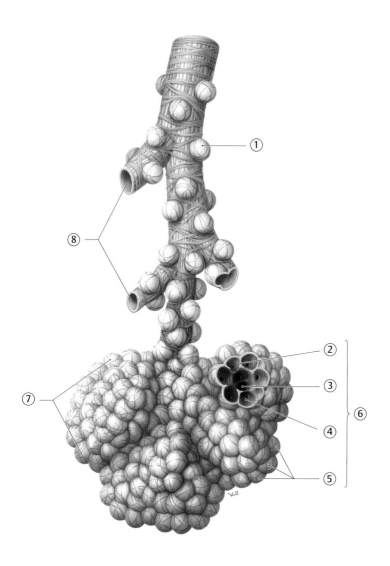

Bronchial Tree: Respiratory Portion

1. pulmonary alveolus
2. interalveolar septum
3. alveolar duct
4. alveolus
5. pulmonary alveoli
6. acinus
7. alveolar sac
8. respiratory bronchioles

Fig. 10.13B. From *Atlas of Anatomy, Third Edition*, p. 121.

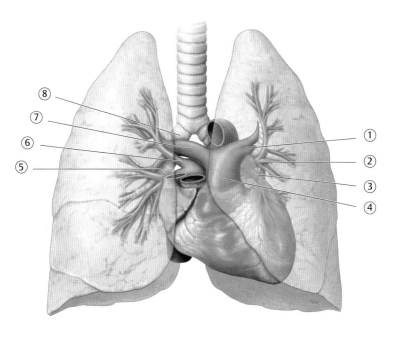

Pulmonary Arteries and Veins

1. left pulmonary a.
2. superior left pulmonary v.
3. inferior left pulmonary v.
4. pulmonary trunk
5. inferior right pulmonary v.
6. superior right pulmonary v.
7. right pulmonary a.
8. right main bronchus

Fig. 10.21C. From *Atlas of Anatomy, Third Edition*, p. 124.

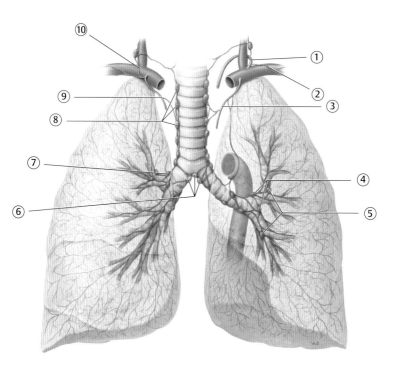

Lymph Nodes and Trunks of the Pleural Cavity

① thoracic duct
② left subclavian trunk
③ left bronchomediastinal trunk
④ bronchopulmonary l.n.
⑤ intrapulmonary l.n.
⑥ inferior tracheobronchial l.n.
⑦ superior tracheobronchial l.n.
⑧ paratracheal l.n.
⑨ right bronchomediastinal trunk
⑩ right jugular trunk

✱ The entire right lung and superior lobe of the left lung normally drain along ipsilateral pathways. However, some lymph from the inferior left lobe may drain to right tracheobronchial nodes and from there follow right-sided channels. This has important implications for metastasis of lung carcinoma.

Fig. 10.29. From *Atlas of Anatomy, Third Edition*, p. 129.

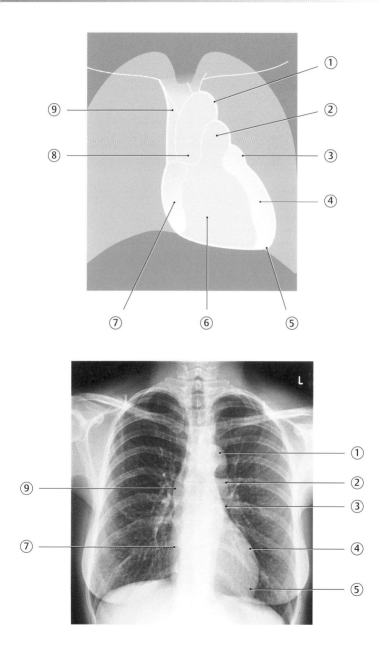

Radiographic Appearance of the Heart, Posteroanterior View

① aortic arch ("aortic knob")
② pulmonary trunk
③ left atrium
④ left ventricle
⑤ cardiac apex
⑥ right ventricle
⑦ right atrium
⑧ aorta (ascending part)
⑨ superior vena cava

Radiographic Appearance of the Heart, Left Lateral View

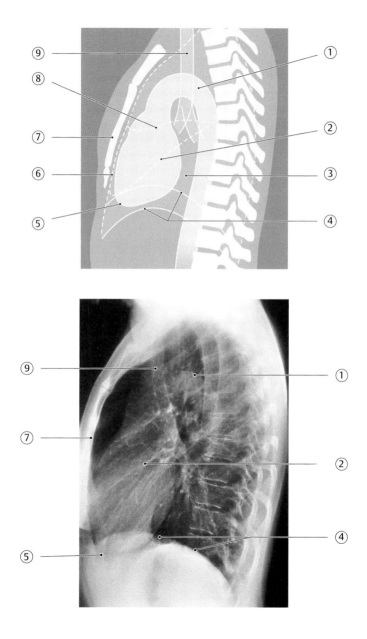

Radiographic Appearance of the Heart, Left Lateral View

①   aortic arch

②   right lung, oblique fissure

③   posterior mediastinum

④   left and right diaphragm leaflets

⑤   cardiac apex

⑥   anterior mediastinum

⑦   sternum, body

⑧   right lung, horizontal fissure

⑨   trachea

Fig. 8.21C,D. From *Atlas of Anatomy, Second Edition*, p. 100.

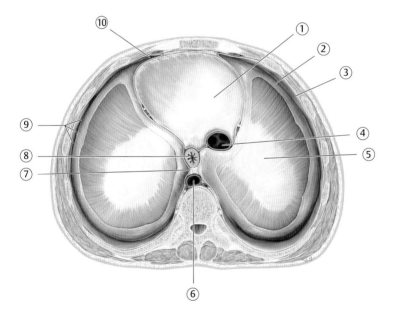

Pleural Recesses

① serous pericardium, parietal layer
② parietal pleura, diaphragmatic part
③ parietal pleura, costal part
④ inferior vena cava
⑤ diaphragm, central tendon
⑥ thoracic aorta
⑦ parietal pleura, mediastinal part
⑧ esophagus
⑨ costodiaphragmatic recess
⑩ costomediastinal recess

Fig. 11.5. From *Atlas of Anatomy, Third Edition*, p. 131.

Abdomen

(Continued)

Abdomen

Regions of the Abdomen

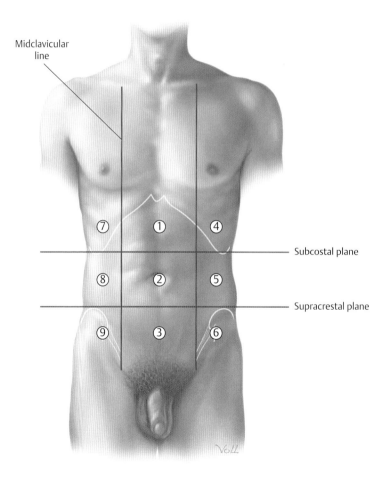

Midclavicular line

Subcostal plane

Supracrestal plane

Regions of the Abdomen

①   epigastric region

②   umbilical region

③   pubic region

④   left hypochondriac region

⑤   left lateral (lumbar) region

⑥   left inguinal region

⑦   right hypochondriac region

⑧   right lateral (lumbar) region

⑨   right inguinal region

Table 12.2. From *Atlas of Anatomy, Third Edition*, p. 141.

Bony Framework of the Abdomen

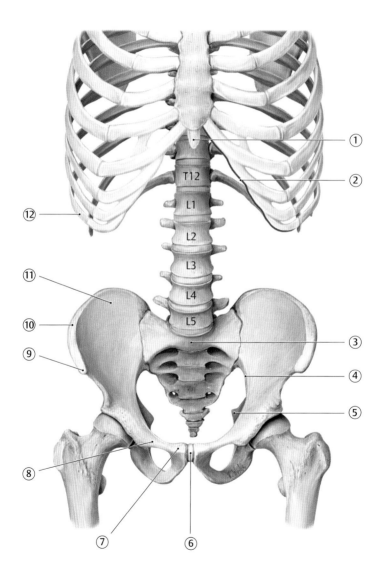

T12
L1
L2
L3
L4
L5

Bony Framework of the Abdomen

① xiphoid process
② costal margin
③ sacral promontory
④ arcuate line
⑤ ischial spine
⑥ pubic symphysis
⑦ pubic tubercle
⑧ superior pubic ramus
⑨ anterior superior iliac spine
⑩ iliac crest
⑪ wing (ala) of sacrum
⑫ 10th rib

Fig. 13.1. From *Atlas of Anatomy, Third Edition*, p. 142.

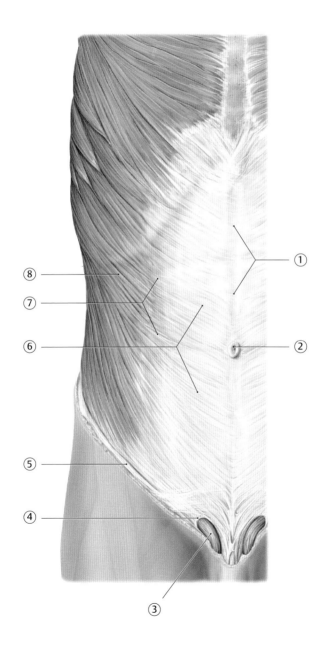

Muscles of the Anterolateral Abdominal Wall I

① linea alba
② umbilicus
③ spermatic cord, cremaster muscle
④ superficial inguinal ring
⑤ inguinal lig.
⑥ rectus sheath, anterior layer
⑦ external oblique aponeurosis
⑧ external oblique

Muscle	Origin	Insertion	Innervation	Action
External oblique	5th–12th ribs (outer surface)	Linea alba, pubic tubercle, anterior iliac crest	Intercostal nn. (T7–T11), subcostal n. (T12)	*Unilateral:* Bends trunk to same side, rotates trunk to opposite side *Bilateral:* Flexes trunk, compresses abdomen, stabilizes pelvis

Fig. 13.4A. From *Atlas of Anatomy, Third Edition*, p. 144.

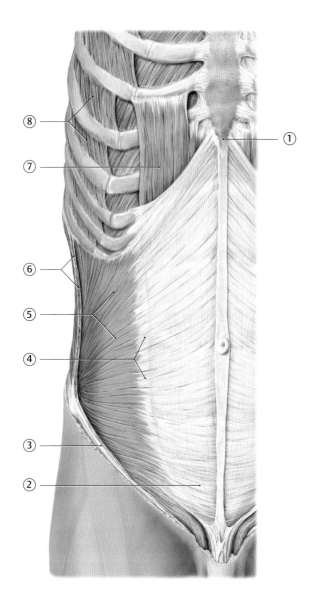

Muscles of the Anterolateral Abdominal Wall II

① xiphoid process
② rectus sheath, anterior layer
③ inguinal lig.
④ internal oblique aponeurosis
⑤ internal oblique
⑥ external oblique
⑦ rectus abdominis
⑧ external intercostals

Muscle	Origin	Insertion	Innervation	Action
Internal oblique	Thoracolumbar fascia (deep layer), iliac crest (intermediate line), anterior superior iliac spine, iliopsoas fascia	10th to12th ribs (lower borders), linea alba (anterior and posterior layers)	Intercostal nn. (T7–T11), subcostal n. (T12) iliohypogastric n., ilioinguinal n.	*Unilateral:* Bends trunk to same side, rotates trunk to opposite side *Bilateral:* Flexes trunk, compresses abdomen, stabilizes pelvis

Fig. 13.4B. From *Atlas of Anatomy, Third Edition*, p. 144.

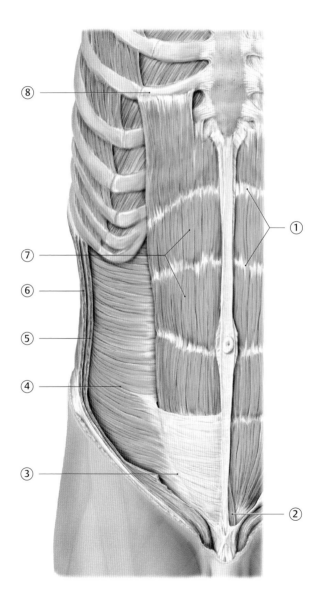

Muscles of the Anterolateral Abdominal Wall III

①   tendinous intersections

②   pyramidalis

③   transverse abdominis aponeurosis

④   transversus abdominis

⑤   internal oblique

⑥   external oblique

⑦   rectus abdominis

⑧   5th costal cartilage

Muscle	Origin	Insertion	Innervation	Action
Anterior abdominal wall muscles				
Rectus abdominis	*Lateral head:* Crest of pubis to pubic tubercle *Medial head:* Anterior region of pubic symphysis	Cartilages of 5th–7th ribs, xiphoid process of sternum	Intercostal nn. (T5–T11) , subcostal n. (T12)	Flexes trunk, compresses abdomen, stabilizes pelvis
Pyramidalis	Pubis (anterior to rectus abdominis)	Linea alba (runs within the rectus sheath)	Subcostal n. (T12)	Tenses linea alba
Anterolateral abdominal wall muscles				
Transversus abdominis	7th–12th costal cartilages (inner surfaces), thoracolumbar fascia (deep layer), iliac crest, anterior superior iliac spine (inner lip), iliopsoas fascia	Linea alba, pubic crest	Intercostal nn. (T7–T11) , subcostal n. (T12) iliohypogastric n., ilioinguinal n.	*Unilateral:* Rotates trunk to same side *Bilateral:* Compresses abdomen

Fig. 13.4C. From *Atlas of Anatomy, Third Edition*, p. 145.

Muscles of the Posterior Abdominal Wall

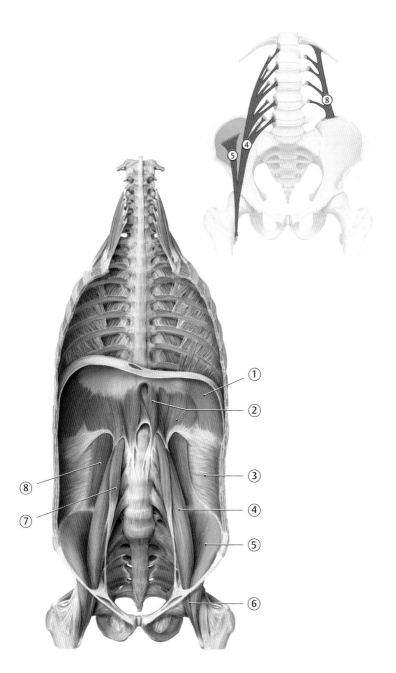

Muscles of the Posterior Abdominal Wall

① diaphragm, costal part
② diaphragm, lumbar part and left crus
③ transversus abdominis
④ psoas major
⑤ iliacus
⑥ Iliopsoas
⑦ psoas minor
⑧ quadratus lumborum

Muscle		Origin	Insertion	Innervation	Action
Psoas minor*		T12, L1 vertebrae and intervertebral disk (lateral surfaces)	Pectineal line, iliopubic ramus, iliac fascia; lowermost fibers may reach inguinal lig.	L1–L2 (L3) spinal nn.	Weak flexor of the trunk
Psoas major	Superficial layer	T12–L4 vertebral bodies and associated intervertebral disks (lateral surfaces)	Femur (lesser trochanter), joint insertion as iliopsoas muscle	L1–L2 (L3) spinal nn.	Hip joint: Flexion and external rotation Lumbar spine (with femur fixed): *Unilateral:* Contraction bends trunk laterally *Bilateral:* Contraction raises trunk from supine position
	Deep layer	L1–L5 (costal processes)			
Iliacus		Iliac fossa		Femoral n. (L2–L4)	
Quadratus lumborum		Iliac crest and iliolumbar lig. (not shown)	12th rib, L1–L4 vertebrae (costal processes)	Subcostal n. (T12), L1–L4 spinal nn.	*Unilateral:* Bends trunk to same side *Bilateral:* Bearing down and expiration, stabilizes 12th rib

*Approximately 50% of the population has this muscle.

Fig. 13.5B, Fig. 13.9. From *Atlas of Anatomy, Third Edition*, p. 146, 148.

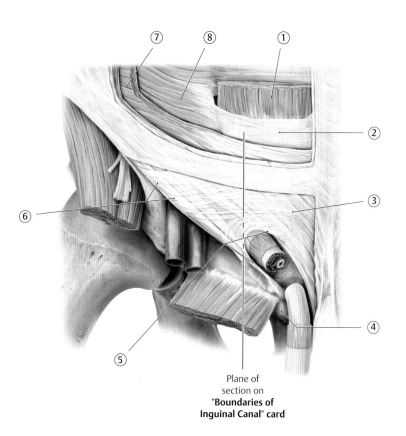

Plane of
section on
**"Boundaries of
Inguinal Canal" card**

Inguinal Region

1. rectus abdominis
2. rectus sheath
3. external oblique aponeurosis
4. pubic tubercle
5. superficial inguinal ring
6. inguinal lig.
7. internal oblique
8. transversus abdominis

Fig. 13.11. From *Atlas of Anatomy, Third Edition*, p. 150.

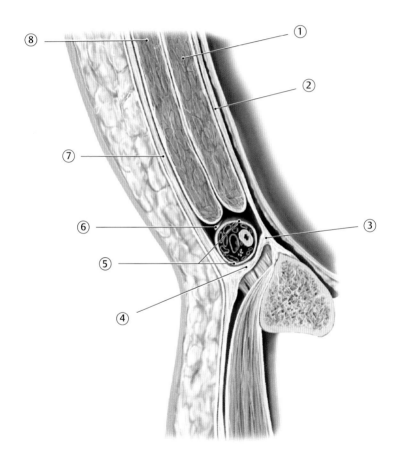

Boundaries of the Inguinal Canal

① transversus abdominis

② transversalis fascia

③ iliopubic tract

④ inguinal lig.

⑤ spermatic cord

⑥ ilioinguinal n.

⑦ external oblique aponeurosis

⑧ internal oblique

Structures of the Inguinal Canal

Structures		Formed by
Wall	Anterior wall	External oblique aponeurosis
	Roof	Internal oblique m.
		Transversus abdominis
	Posterior wall	Transversalis fascia
		Parietal peritoneum
	Floor	Inguinal lig. (densely interwoven fibers of the lower external oblique aponeurosis and adjacent fascia lata of thigh)
Openings	Superficial inguinal ring	Opening in external oblique aponeurosis; bounded by medial and lateral crus, intercrural fibers, and reflected inguinal lig.
	Deep inguinal ring	Outpouching of the transversalis fascia lateral to the lateral umbilical fold (inferior epigastric vessels)
Sagittal section through plane on **"Inguinal Region" card**		

Table 13.3. From *Atlas of Anatomy, Third Edition*, p. 151.

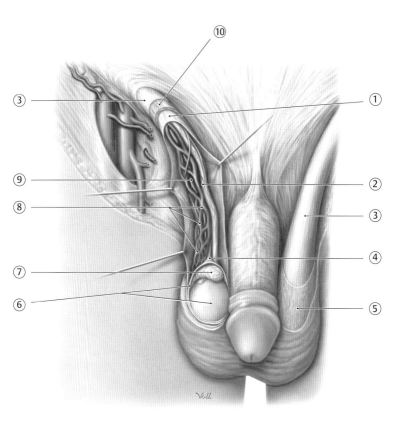

Scrotum and Spermatic Cord

① internal spermatic fascia

② ductus deferens

③ external spermatic fascia

④ processus vaginalis (obliterated)

⑤ tunica dartos

⑥ tunica vaginalis, parietal and visceral layers

⑦ epididymis

⑧ pampiniform plexus (testicular vv.)

⑨ testicular a.

⑩ cremasteric fascia and cremasteric m.

Structures of the Inguinal Canal	
Covering layer	**Derived from**
Scrotal skin	Abdominal skin
Tunica dartos	Dartos fascia and m.
External spermatic fascia	External oblique fascia
Cremaster m. and/or cremasteric fascia	Internal oblique
Internal spermatic fascia	Transversalis fascia
Tunica vaginalis, parietal layer	Peritoneum
Tunica vaginalis, visceral layer	
Note: The transversus abdominis has no contribution to the spermatic cord or covering of the testis.	

Fig. 13.14. From *Atlas of Anatomy, Third Edition*, p. 152.

Testis and Epididymis

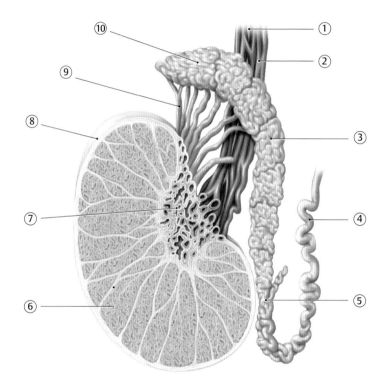

What is the function of the epididymis?

Testis and Epididymis

1. testicular a.
2. pampiniform plexus
3. epididymis, body
4. ductus deferens
5. epididymis, tail
6. lobule
7. rete testis in mediastinum testes
8. tunica albuginea
9. efferent ductules
10. epididymis, head

The epididymis, a highly coiled tubule that hugs the back of the testis, is the site for sperm maturation and storage. Continuous distally with the ductus deferens, it is part of the male ductal system that transports sperm from the testis to the genital structures in the pelvis.

Fig. 13.16C. From *Atlas of Anatomy, Third Edition*, p. 153.

Inferior Anterior Abdominal Wall

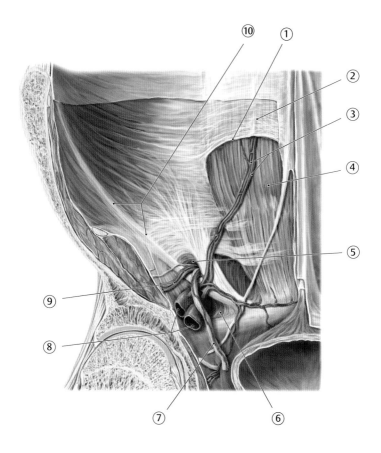

What is the deep inguinal ring?

Inferior Anterior Abdominal Wall

1. arcuate line
2. rectus sheath, posterior layer
3. inferior epigastric a. and v.
4. rectus abdominis
5. deep inguinal ring
6. femoral ring
7. ductus deferens
8. external iliac a. and v.
9. testicular a. and v.
10. iliopubic tract

⚠ The deep inguinal ring lies in the lateral inguinal fossa and is formed by an evagination of the transversalis fascia into the inguinal canal. In the male it is traversed by the ductus deferens and testicular vessels and nerves that make up the spermatic cord.

Fig. 13.18. From *Atlas of Anatomy, Third Edition*, p. 155.

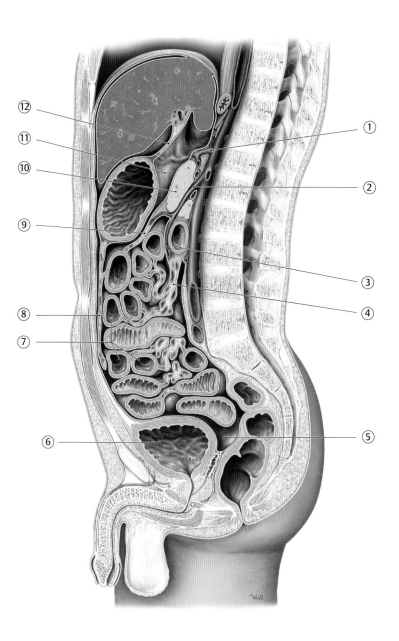

Peritoneal Relations of Abdominopelvic Organs

①   celiac trunk

②   superior mesenteric a.

③   duodenum, horizontal part

④   mesentery

⑤   rectovesical pouch

⑥   urinary bladder

⑦   jejunum and ileum

⑧   greater omentum

⑨   transverse mesocolon

⑩   pancreas, neck

⑪   omental bursa (lesser sac)

⑫   hepatogastric lig. (lesser omentum)

Fig. 14.2. From *Atlas of Anatomy, Third Edition*, p. 157.

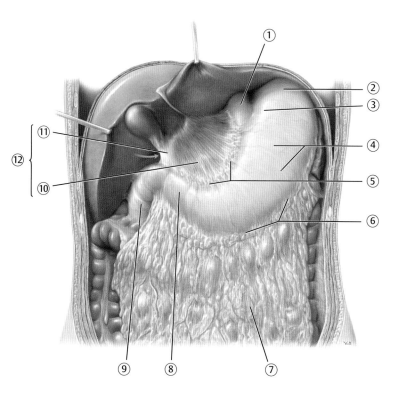

Stomach In Situ

1. esophagus
2. stomach, fundus
3. stomach, cardia
4. stomach body
5. lesser curvature
6. greater curvature
7. greater omentum
8. pyloric canal
9. duodenum
10. hepatogastric lig.
11. hepatoduodenal lig.
12. lesser omentum

Fig. 15.4. From *Atlas of Anatomy, Third Edition*, p. 165.

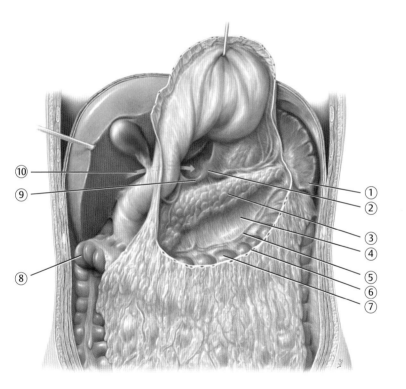

⑩ ⑨ ⑧

① ② ③ ④ ⑤ ⑥ ⑦

What are the boundaries of the omental foramen?

Omental Bursa In Situ

① spleen
② celiac trunk
③ pancreas
④ transverse mesocolon
⑤ middle colic a. and v.
⑥ gastrocolic lig.
⑦ transverse colon
⑧ right colic flexure
⑨ common hepatic a.
⑩ omental foramen

❗ The omental (epiploic) foramen, the opening between the greater sac and lesser sac (omental bursa), is bounded anteriorly by the portal v., proper hepatic a., and bile duct; posteriorly by the inferior vena cava and left crus of the diaphragm; superiorly by the liver; and inferiorly by the duodenum.

Fig. 14.6. From *Atlas of Anatomy, Third Edition*, p. 161.

Mesenteries of the Peritoneal Cavity

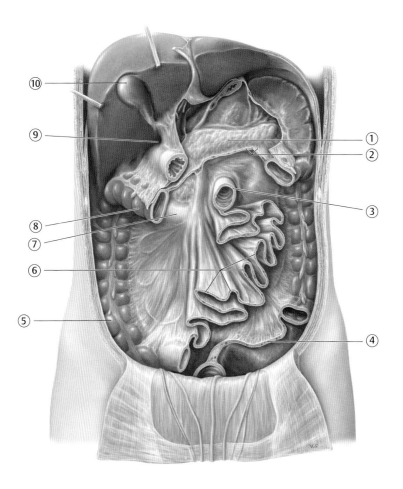

❓ Which parts of the small and large intestines are associated with a mesentery?

Mesenteries of the Peritoneal Cavity

① pancreas

② transverse mesocolon, root

③ duodenojejunal flexure

④ sigmoid mesocolon

⑤ ascending colon

⑥ mesentery

⑦ duodenum, horizontal part

⑧ transverse colon

⑨ omental foramen

⑩ gallbladder

⚠ Most of the small intestine is suspended by mesenteries—the proximal part of the duodenum by the lesser omentum, and the jejunum and ileum by the mesentery (of the small bowel). Of the four parts of the large intestine, only the transverse and sigmoid colons are suspended by mesenteries, the transverse and sigmoid mesocolons.

Fig. 14.7. From *Atlas of Anatomy, Third Edition*, p. 162.

Duodenum

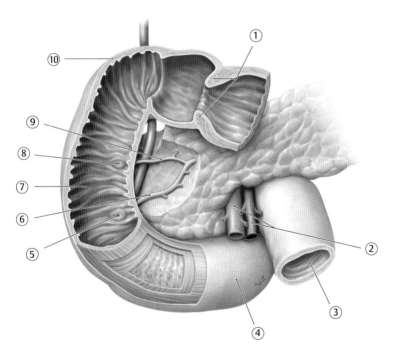

Duodenum

1. pyloric sphincter
2. superior mesenteric a. and v.
3. jejunum
4. duodenum, horizontal part
5. major duodenal papilla
6. main pancreatic duct
7. duodenum, descending part
8. minor duodenal papilla
9. accessory pancreatic duct
10. duodenum, superior part

Fig. 15.7. From *Atlas of Anatomy, Third Edition*, p. 166.

Large Intestine

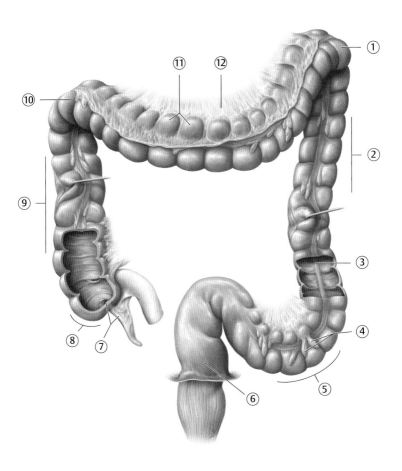

Name three gross features of the large intestine that distinguish it from the small intestine.

Large Intestine

1. left colic (splenic) flexure
2. descending colon
3. tenia coli
4. epiploic appendices
5. sigmoid colon
6. rectum
7. vermiform appendix (with orifice)
8. cecum
9. ascending colon
10. right colic (hepatic) flexure
11. haustra
12. transverse mesocolon

Features of the large intestine that are lacking in the small intestine include haustra, tenia coli, and epiploic appendages.

Fig. 15.15. From *Atlas of Anatomy, Third Edition*, p. 170.

Surfaces of the Liver, Anterior View

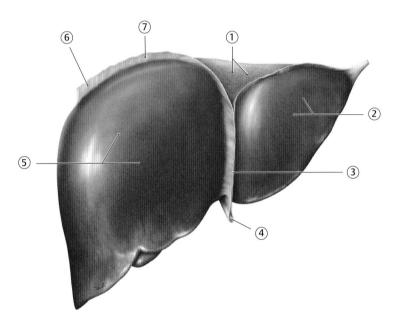

Surfaces of the Liver, Anterior View

①   bare area (diaphragmatic surface of liver)

②   left lobe

③   falciform lig.

④   round lig.

⑤   right lobe

⑥   right triangular lig.

⑦   coronary lig.

Fig. 15.22A. From *Atlas of Anatomy, Third Edition*, p. 174.

Surfaces of the Liver, Inferior View

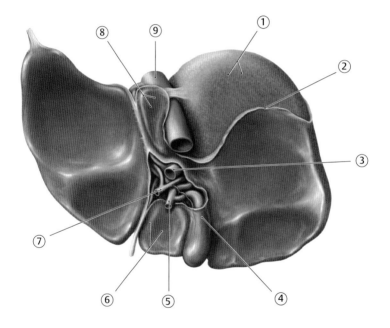

🖼 What is the bare area of the liver?

Surfaces of the Liver, Inferior View

① bare area

② coronary lig.

③ portal v.

④ gallbladder

⑤ bile duct

⑥ quadrate lobe

⑦ proper hepatic a.

⑧ caudate lobe

⑨ inferior vena cava

! The bare area on the superior and posterior surfaces of the liver lacks a peritoneal covering and therefore is in direct contact with the diaphragm. The area is defined by the coronary and triangular ligs., which are single-layer peritoneal reflections.

Fig. 15.22B. From *Atlas of Anatomy, Third Edition*, p. 174.

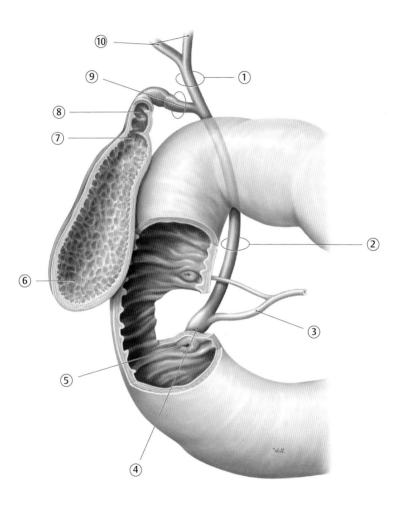

Extrahepatic Bile Ducts

① common hepatic duct
② bile duct
③ pancreatic duct
④ hepatopancreatic ampulla
⑤ major duodenal papilla
⑥ fundus of gallbladder
⑦ infundibulum of gallbladder
⑧ neck of gallbladder
⑨ cystic duct
⑩ right and left hepatic ducts

Gallstones are concretions of cholesterol that lodge within the biliary tree. Although they may be asymptomatic, they can also cause severe pain. When lodged in the hepatopancreatic ampulla, they can obstruct the flow of bile and pancreatic secretions into the duodenum, leading to pancreatitis.

Fig. 15.27. From *Atlas of Anatomy, Third Edition*, p. 176.

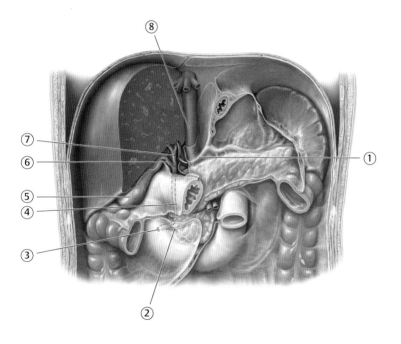

Biliary Tract In Situ

1. common hepatic a.
2. pancreatic duct
3. hepatopancreatic duct (opening on major duodenal papilla)
4. bile duct
5. gallbladder
6. cystic duct
7. common hepatic duct
8. inferior vena cava

Fig. 15.28. From *Atlas of Anatomy, Third Edition*, p. 177.

Pancreas

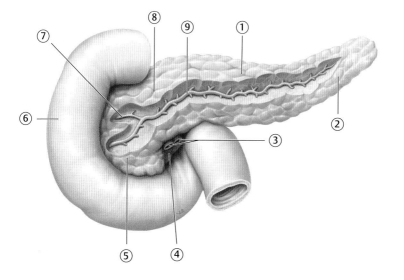

Pancreas

① pancreas, body
② pancreas, tail
③ superior mesenteric a. and v.
④ pancreas, uncinate process
⑤ pancreas, head
⑥ duodenum, descending part
⑦ accessory pancreatic duct
⑧ pancreas, neck
⑨ pancreatic duct

Fig. 15.30. From *Atlas of Anatomy, Third Edition*, p. 178.

Kidney I

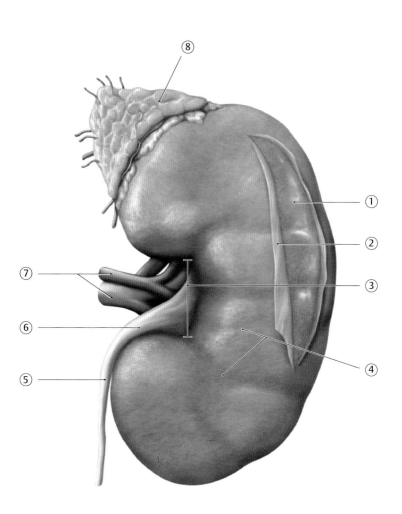

Describe the layers that surround the kidney.

Kidney I

① renal cortex
② fibrous capsule
③ renal hilum
④ posterior surface
⑤ right ureter
⑥ renal pelvis
⑦ right renal a. and v.
⑧ right suprarenal gland

❗ Each kidney, with its associated suprarenal gland and hilar structures, is enveloped by a layer of perirenal fat, which is contained by the renal (Gerota) fascia. Pararenal fat lies outside this layer.

Fig. 15.38B. From *Atlas of Anatomy, Third Edition*, p. 182.

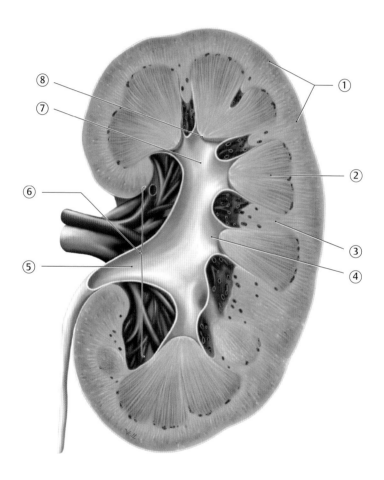

Kidney II

1. renal cortex
2. renal pyramid
3. renal column
4. minor calyx
5. renal pelvis
6. renal sinus
7. major calyx
8. renal papilla

Fig. 15.38D. From *Atlas of Anatomy, Third Edition*, p. 182.

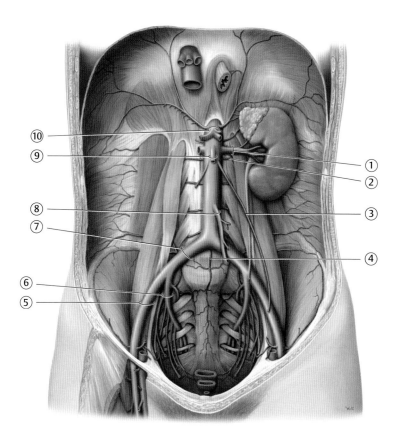

Abdominal Aorta

① left renal a.

② left 1st lumbar a.

③ left ovarian a.

④ median sacral a.

⑤ right external iliac a.

⑥ right internal iliac a.

⑦ right common iliac a.

⑧ inferior mesenteric a.

⑨ superior mesenteric a.

⑩ celiac trunk

Branches of the Abdominal Aorta

The abdominal aorta gives rise to three major unpaired trunks (bold) and the unpaired median sacral artery, as well as six paired branches.

Branch from abdominal aorta	Branches		
Inferior phrenic aa. (paired)	Superior suprarenal aa.		
Celiac trunk	Left gastric a.		
	Splenic a.		
	Common hepatic a.	Proper hepatic a.	
		Right gastric a.	
		Gastroduodenal a.	
Middle suprarenal aa. (paired)			
Superior mesenteric a.			
Renal aa. (paired)	Inferior suprarenal aa.		
Lumbar aa. (1st through 4th, paired)			
Testicular/ovarian aa. (paired)			
Inferior mesenteric a.			
Common iliac aa. (paired)	External iliac a.		
	Internal iliac a.		
Median sacral a.			

Fig. 16.7. From *Atlas of Anatomy, Third Edition*, p. 186.

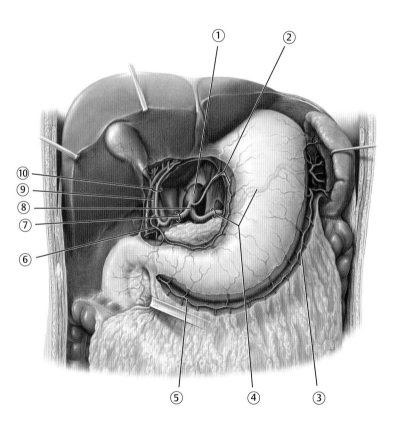

Celiac trunk I

1. abdominal aorta
2. left gastric a.
3. left gastro-omental a.
4. splenic a.
5. right gastro-omental a.
6. right gastric a.
7. common hepatic a.
8. celiac trunk
9. portal v.
10. proper hepatic a.

Fig. 16.9. From *Atlas of Anatomy, Third Edition*, p. 188.

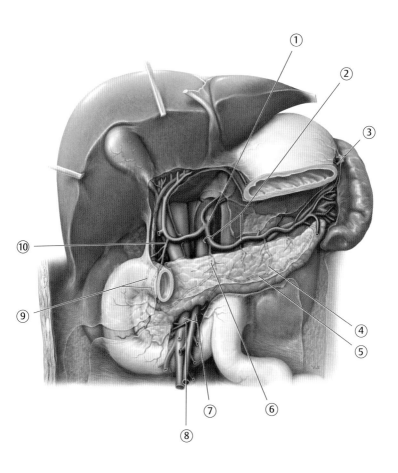

Celiac Trunk II

①   celiac trunk

②   splenic a.

③   short gastric aa.

④   great pancreatic a.

⑤   inferior pancreatic a.

⑥   dorsal pancreatic a.

⑦   superior mesenteric a. and v.

⑧   inferior pancreaticoduodenal a.

⑨   anterior and posterior superior pancreaticoduodenal aa.

⑩   gastroduodenal a.

❄ The pancreaticoduodenal arcade is an important anastomosis between branches of the superior mesenteric a. and the gastroduodenal a., a branch of the celiac trunk.

Fig. 16.10. From *Atlas of Anatomy, Third Edition*, p. 189.

Superior Mesenteric Artery

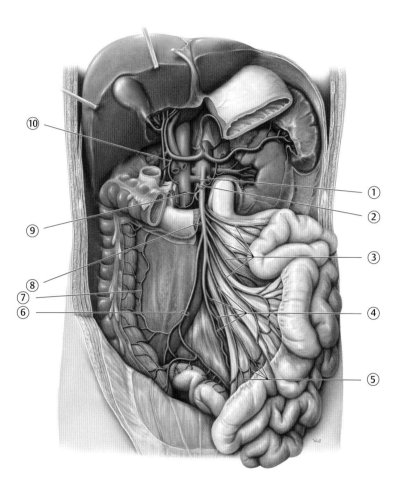

The superior mesenteric a. supplies structures of the midgut. What does this include?

Superior Mesenteric Artery

① superior mesenteric a.

② middle colic a.

③ jejunal aa.

④ ileal aa.

⑤ vasa recta

⑥ ileocolic a.

⑦ marginal a.

⑧ right colic a.

⑨ inferior pancreaticoduodenal a., anterior and posterior branches

⑩ gastroduodenal a.

⚠ The midgut supplied by the superior mesenteric a. extends from the middle portion of the duodenum to the distal two thirds of the transverse colon.

Fig. 16.11. From *Atlas of Anatomy, Third Edition*, p. 190.

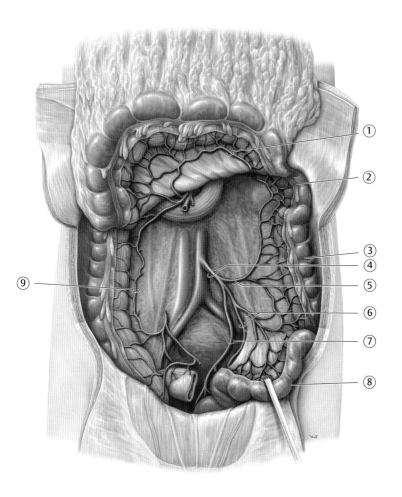

Inferior Mesenteric Artery

① marginal a.
② left colic (splenic) flexure
③ descending colon
④ inferior mesenteric a.
⑤ left colic a.
⑥ sigmoid aa.
⑦ superior rectal a.
⑧ sigmoid colon
⑨ marginal a.

Fig. 16.12. From *Atlas of Anatomy, Third Edition*, p. 191.

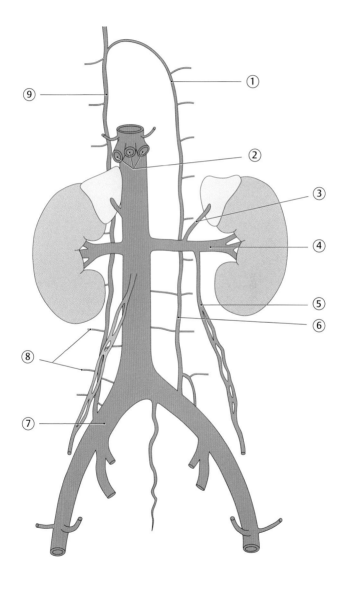

Tributaries of the Inferior Vena Cava

①   hemiazygos v.

②   hepatic vv.

③   left suprarenal v.

④   left renal v.

⑤   left testicular/ovarian v.

⑥   left ascending lumbar v.

⑦   right common iliac v.

⑧   lumbar vv.

⑨   azygos v.

Tributaries of the Inferior Vena Cava
Inferior phrenic vv. (paired)
Hepatic vv. (3)
Suprarenal vv. (the right vein is a direct tributary)
Renal vv. (paired)
Testicular/ovarian vv. (the right vein is a direct tributary)
Ascending lumbar vv. (paired), not direct tributaries
Lumbar vv.
Common iliac vv. (paired)
Median sacral v.

Table 16.2. From *Atlas of Anatomy, Third Edition*, p. 192.

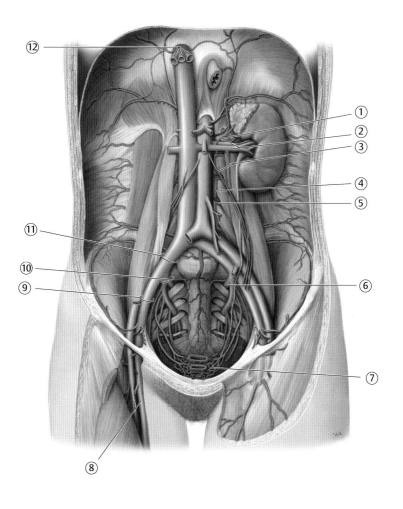

Inferior Vena Cava

① left suprarenal v.
② left renal a. and v.
③ left ovarian a. and v.
④ left ascending lumbar v.
⑤ left 3rd lumbar v.
⑥ left superior gluteal v.
⑦ uterine venous plexus
⑧ femoral a. and v.
⑨ right external iliac v.
⑩ right internal iliac v.
⑪ right common iliac v.
⑫ hepatic vv.

Fig. 16.16. From *Atlas of Anatomy, Third Edition*, p. 194.

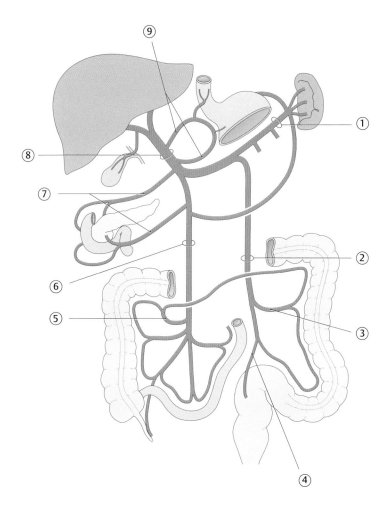

Portal Vein Distribution

①   splenic v.

②   inferior mesenteric v.

③   left colic v.

④   superior rectal v.

⑤   middle colic v.

⑥   superior mesenteric v.

⑦   pancreaticoduodenal vv.

⑧   portal v.

⑨   gastric vv.

Fig. 16.15B. From *Atlas of Anatomy, Third Edition*, p. 193.

Portal Vein

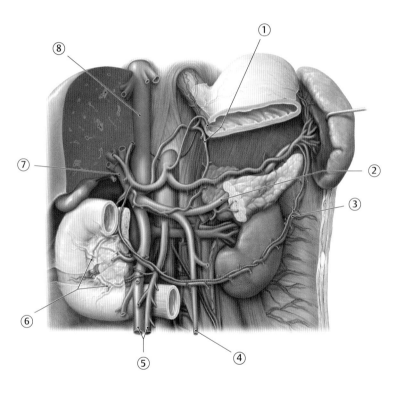

🔲 Which organs of the abdomen are drained by the hepatic portal system?

Portal Vein

① left gastric a. and v.

② splenic v.

③ left gastro-omental a. and v.

④ inferior mesenteric v.

⑤ superior mesenteric v.

⑥ pancreaticoduodenal v.

⑦ portal v.

⑧ inferior vena cava

❗ The hepatic portal system drains the gastrointestinal tract from the lower esophagus to the upper part of the rectum. It also drains the liver, gallbladder, pancreas, and spleen.

Fig. 16.19. From *Atlas of Anatomy, Third Edition*, p. 197.

Lymph Nodes of the Posterior Abdominal Wall

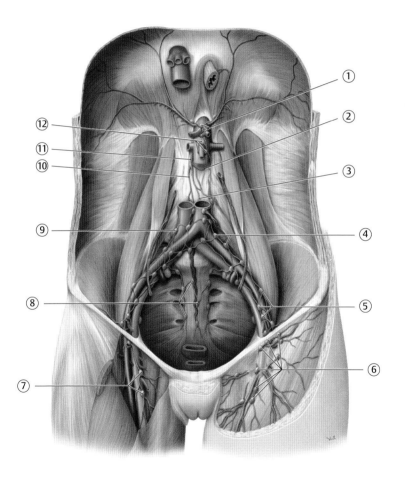

Lymph Nodes of the Posterior Abdominal Wall

① celiac l.n.
② intestinal trunk
③ retroaortic l.n.
④ common iliac l.n.
⑤ external iliac l.n.
⑥ superficial inguinal l.n. (horizontal and vertical groups)
⑦ deep inguinal l.n.
⑧ sacral l.n.
⑨ right lateral caval l.n.
⑩ right lumbar trunk
⑪ cisterna chyli
⑫ superior mesenteric l.n.

✱ Lymph that collects in the cisterna chyli drains to the thoracic duct, which passes superiorly through the thorax into the root of the neck, where it empties into the left jugulosubclavian junction.

Fig. 16.24. From *Atlas of Anatomy, Third Edition*, p. 202.

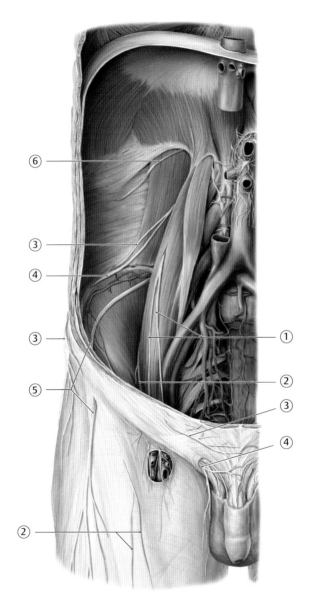

Spinal nerves from which vertebral levels contribute to the lumbar plexus?

Nerves of the Lumbar Plexus

① genitofemoral n., genital and femoral branches
② femoral n.
③ iliohypogastric n.
④ ilioinguinal n.
⑤ lateral femoral cutaneous n.
⑥ subcostal n.

! The lumbar plexus is formed by the anterior rami of spinal nerves L1–L4.

Fig. 16.37. From *Atlas of Anatomy, Third Edition*, p. 209.

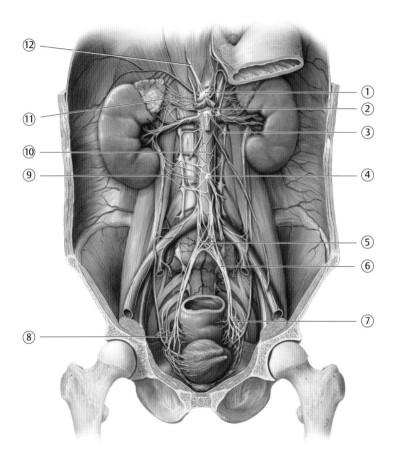

Autonomic Plexuses in the Abdomen and Pelvis

① celiac ganglion
② aorticorenal ganglia
③ superior mesenteric ganglion
④ inferior mesenteric ganglion
⑤ superior hypogastric plexus
⑥ left hypogastric n.
⑦ inferior hypogastric plexus
⑧ pelvic splanchnic nn.
⑨ sympathetic trunk
⑩ intermesenteric plexus
⑪ suprarenal plexus
⑫ right greater splanchnic n.

Fig. 16.42. From *Atlas of Anatomy, Third Edition*, p. 215.

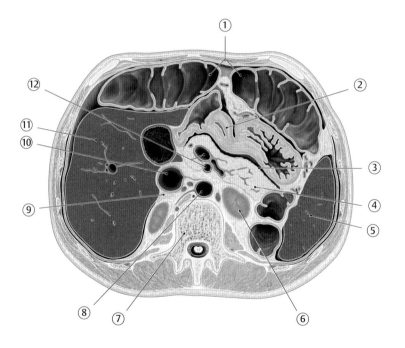

Axial Section of the Abdomen

1. transverse colon
2. pylorus of the stomach
3. omental bursa
4. pancreas
5. spleen
6. left kidney
7. L1 vertebra
8. abdominal aorta
9. right suprarenal gland
10. inferior vena cava
11. gallbladder
12. superior mesenteric a. and v.

Fig. 17.1B. From *Atlas of Anatomy, Third Edition*, p. 218.

Pelvis & Perineum

Hip (Coxal) Bone

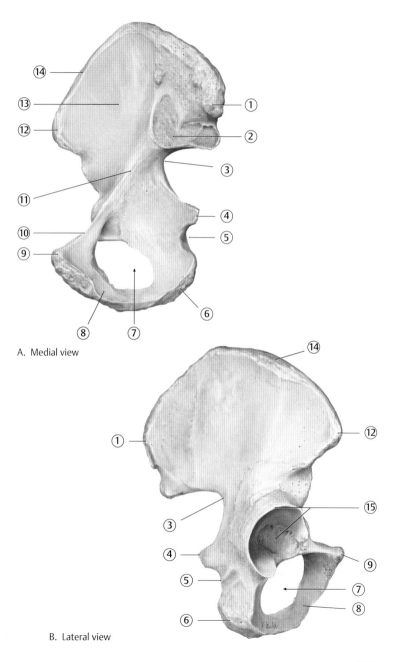

A. Medial view

B. Lateral view

Hip (Coxal) Bone

1. posterior superior iliac spine
2. auricular surface of ilium
3. greater sciatic notch
4. ischial spine
5. lesser sciatic notch
6. ischial tuberosity
7. obturator foramen
8. inferior pubic ramus
9. pubic tubercle
10. pectineal line
11. arcuate line
12. anterior superior iliac spine
13. iliac fossa
14. iliac crest
15. acetabular rim and fossa

Fig. 19.2, Fig. 19.4. From *Atlas of Anatomy, Third Edition*, p. 228–229.

Female Bony Pelvis

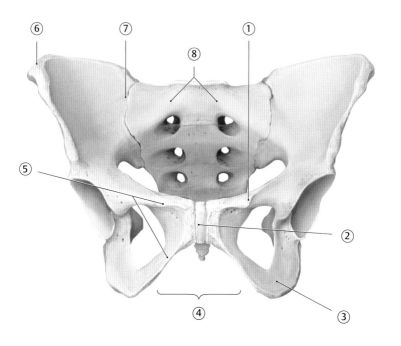

Female Bony Pelvis

1. pubic tubercle
2. pubic symphysis
3. ischial ramus
4. pubic arch
5. superior and inferior pubic rami
6. iliac crest
7. sacroiliac joint
8. sacrum

Fig. 19.5A. From *Atlas of Anatomy, Third Edition*, p. 230.

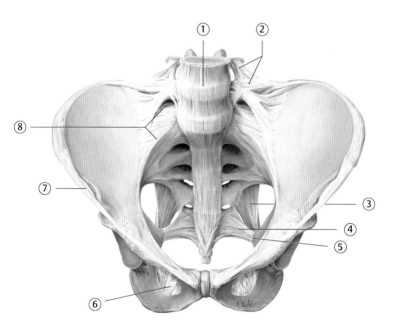

Ligaments of the Pelvis I, Anterior View

① anterior longitudinal lig.
② Iliolumbar lig.
③ sacrotuberous lig.
④ sacrospinous lig.
⑤ ischial spine
⑥ obturator membrane
⑦ inguinal lig.
⑧ anterior sacroiliac ligs.

Fig. 19.10A. From *Atlas of Anatomy, Third Edition*, p. 234.

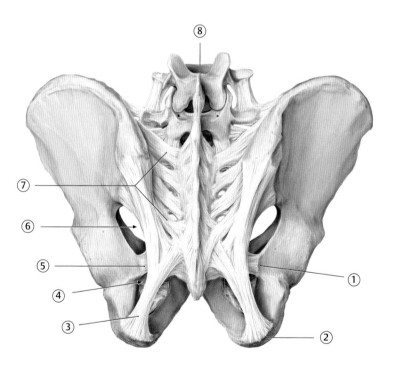

Ligaments of the Pelvis II, Posterior View

① ischial spine
② ischial tuberosity
③ sacrotuberous lig.
④ lesser sciatic foramen
⑤ sacrospinous lig.
⑥ greater sciatic foramen
⑦ posterior sacroiliac ligs.
⑧ L4 spinous process

Fig. 19.10B. From *Atlas of Anatomy, Third Edition*, p. 234.

Ligaments of the Pelvis III, Medial View

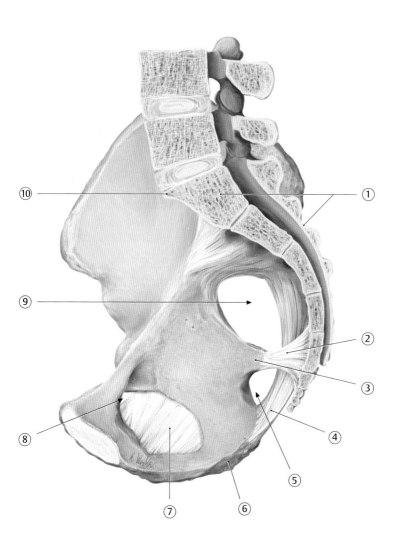

🔲 Which neurovascular bundle passes through both the greater and lesser sciatic foramina?

Ligaments of the Pelvis III, Medial View

①   sacrum

②   sacrospinous lig.

③   ischial spine

④   sacrotuberous lig.

⑤   lesser sciatic foramen

⑥   ischial tuberosity

⑦   obturator membrane

⑧   obturator canal

⑨   greater sciatic foramen

⑩   promontory

❗ The internal pudendal a. and v. and the pudendal n. pass through both foramina. They exit the pelvis through the greater sciatic foramen and enter the perineum through the lesser sciatic foramen.

Fig. 19.11A. From *Atlas of Anatomy, Third Edition*, p. 235.

Muscles of the Pelvic Diaphragm

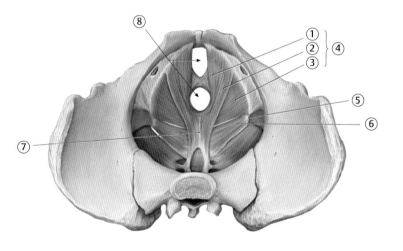

Muscles of the Pelvic Diaphragm

①   puborectalis

②   pubococcygeus

③   iliococcygeus

④   levator ani

⑤   ischial spine

⑥   coccygeus

⑦   anococcygeal Raphe

⑧   urogenital hiatus

Muscle		Origin	Insertion	Innervation	Action
Levator ani	Puborectalis	Superior pubic ramus (both sides of pubic symphysis)	Anococcygeal lig.	Nerve to levator ani (S4), inferior rectal n.	Pelvic diaphragm: Supports pelvic viscera
	Pubococcygeus	Pubis (lateral to origin of puborectalis)	Anococcygeal lig., coccyx		
	Iliococcygeus	Internal obturator fascia of levator ani (tendinous arch)			
Coccygeus		Lateral surface of coccyx and S5 segment	Ischial spine	Direct branches from sacral plexus (S4–S5)	Supports pelvic viscera, flexes coccyx

Fig. 19.13A. From *Atlas of Anatomy, Third Edition*, p. 236.

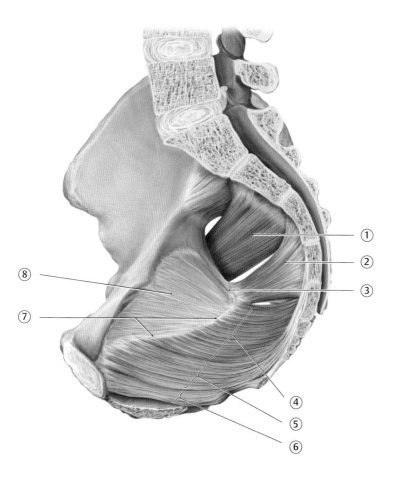

Muscles of the Pelvic Walls

① piriformis

② coccygeus

③ ischial spine

④ iliococcygeus

⑤ pubococcygeus

⑥ puborectalis

⑦ tendinous arch of levator ani

⑧ obturator internus fascia

	Origin	Insertion	Innervation	Action
Piriformis*	Sacrum (pelvic surface)	Femur (apex of greater trochanter)	Direct branches from sacral plexus (S1–S2)	Hip joint: External rotation, stabilization, and abduction of flexed hip
Obturator internus*	Obturator membrane and bony boundaries (inner surface)	Femur (greater trochanter, medial surface)	Direct branches from sacral plexus (L5–S1)	Hip joint: External rotation and abduction of flexed hip
*The piriformis and obturator internus are considered muscles of the hip.				

Fig. 19.13C. From *Atlas of Anatomy, Third Edition*, p. 236.

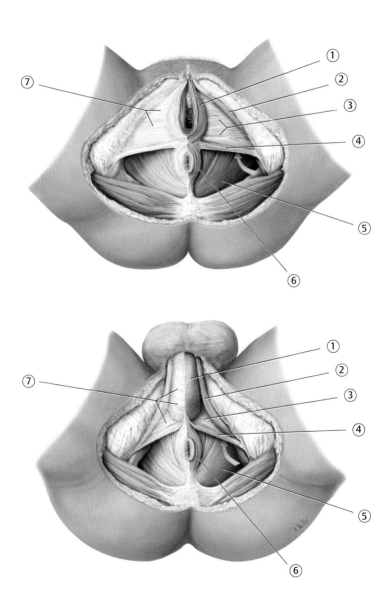

Muscles of the Perineum I

① bulbospongiosus
② ischiocavernosus
③ perineal membrane
④ superficial transverse perineal
⑤ levator ani
⑥ external anal sphincter
⑦ superficial perineal (Colles) fascia

Muscle	Origin	Insertion	Innervation	Action
Ischiocavernosus	Ischial ramus	Crus of clitoris or penis	Pudendal n. (S2–S4)	Maintains erection by squeezing blood into corpus cavernosum of clitoris or penis
Bulbospongiosus	Runs anteriorly from perineal body to clitoris (females) or penile raphe (males)			Females: Compresses greater vestibular gland Males: Assists in erection
Superficial transverse perineal	Ischial ramus	Perineal body		Helps hold perineal body in median plane, holds the pelvic organs in place, and supports visceral canals through the muscles of the perineum

Fig. 19.14A,B. From *Atlas of Anatomy, Third Edition*, p. 237.

Muscles of the Perineum II

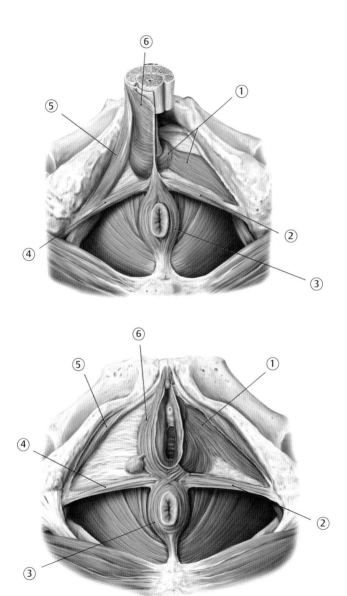

Muscles of the Perineum II

① external urethral sphincter

② deep transverse perineal

③ external anal sphincter

④ superficial transverse perineal

⑤ ischiocavernosus

⑥ bulbospongiosus

Muscle	Origin	Insertion	Innervation	Action
Deep transverse perineal*	Inferior pubic ramus, ischial ramus	Crus of clitoris or penis	Pudendal n. (S2–S4)	Helps hold perineal body in median plane, holds the pelvic organs in place, and supports visceral canals through the muscles of the perineum
External urethral sphincter		Encircles urethra (division of deep transverse perineal muscle), in males ascends anteriorly to neck of the bladder; in females, some fibers surround the vagina as the urethrovaginal sphincter		Closes urethra
External anal sphincter		Encircles anus (runs posteriorly from perineal body to anococcygeal lig.)		Closes anus
*Typically, the deep transverse perineal is not developed in females and is replaced by smooth muscle tissue. When developed, it provides dynamic support to the pelvic organs.				

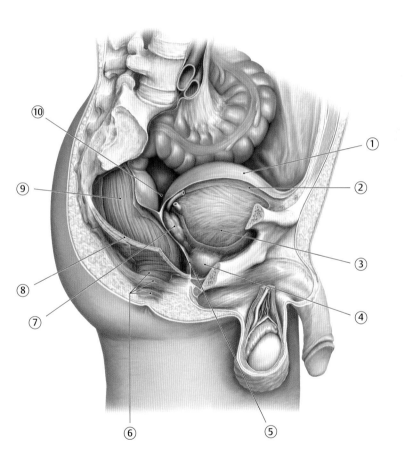

What is the function of the seminal glands?

Male Pelvis

1. visceral peritoneum on bladder
2. visceral pelvic fascia on bladder
3. urinary bladder
4. prostate
5. rectoprostatic fascia
6. external anal sphincter
7. right seminal gland
8. levator ani
9. rectum
10. rectovesical pouch

! The seminal glands are paired convoluted tubules that produce 70% of the seminal fluid.

Fig. 20.1. From *Atlas of Anatomy, Third Edition*, p. 240.

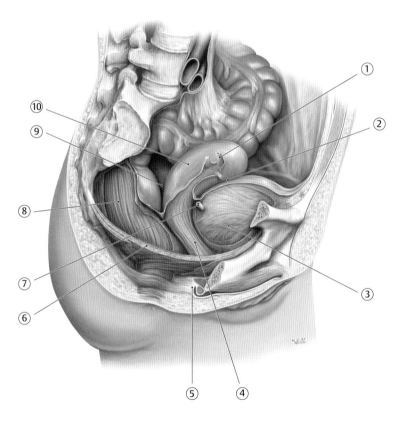

Female Pelvis

1. uterine tube
2. vesicouterine pouch
3. urinary bladder
4. vagina
5. perineal body
6. levator ani
7. right ureter
8. rectum
9. rectouterine pouch
10. uterus

Fig. 20.2. From *Atlas of Anatomy, Third Edition*, p. 241.

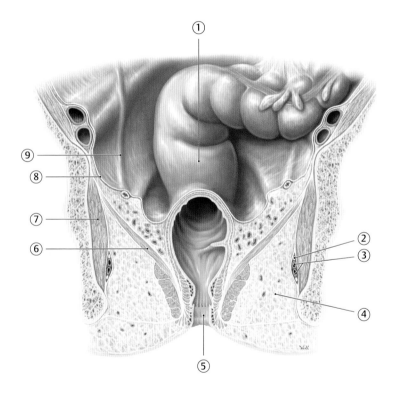

Rectum In Situ

①   rectum

②   pudendal n.

③   internal pudendal a. and v.

④   ischioanal fossa

⑤   anal canal

⑥   levator ani

⑦   obturator internus

⑧   parietal peritoneum

⑨   ureter

Fig. 21.3. From *Atlas of Anatomy, Third Edition*, p. 246.

Rectum and Anal Canal

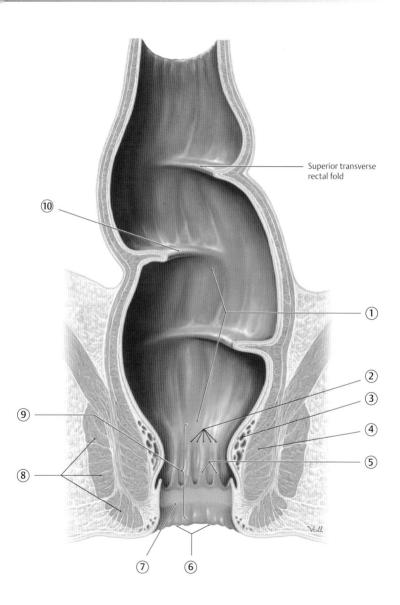

Superior transverse rectal fold

The dentate (pectinate) line is an irregular line formed at the base of the anal columns. How does innervation of the anal canal differ above and below this line?

Rectum and Anal Canal

①   rectal ampulla

②   anorectal junction

③   hemorrhoidal plexus

④   internal anal sphincter

⑤   anal columns

⑥   anus

⑦   anocutaneous line

⑧   external anal sphincter, deep, superficial, and subcutaneous parts

⑨   anal canal

⚠ Above the dentate (pectinate) line, the anal canal is innervated by autonomic fibers that regulate the contraction and relaxation of the internal sphincter. Visceral sensory fibers convey sensations of stretching but not of pain. Below this line, the anal canal is innervated by somatic fibers that regulate contraction of the external sphincter. Somatic sensory fibers transmit sensations of pain, touch, and temperature.

Fig. 21.4. From *Atlas of Anatomy, Third Edition*, p. 247.

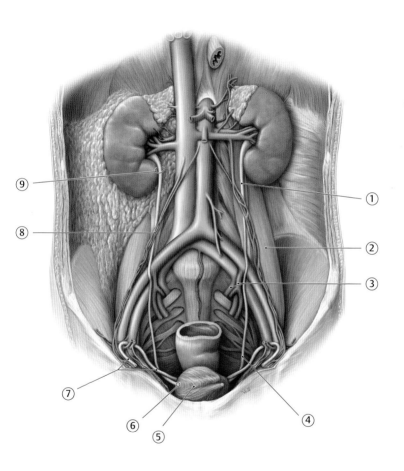

Along the course of the ureter, renal calculi (kidney stones) may become lodged at sites where the ureter narrows or is compressed by adjacent structures. Where are the most common sites for this?

Ureters In Situ

① ureter, abdominal part

② psoas major

③ left internal iliac a. and v.

④ ureter, pelvic part

⑤ urinary bladder

⑥ ureterovesical junction

⑦ right ductus deferens

⑧ right gonadal a. and v.

⑨ ureteropelvic junction

❗ Anatomic constrictions of the ureter commonly occur at the ureteropelvic junction, where the renal pelvis narrows; at the pelvic brim, where the ureter crosses the external iliac artery and vein; and at the ureterovesical junction, where the ureter passes through the wall of the bladder.

Fig. 21.5. From *Atlas of Anatomy, Third Edition*, p. 248.

Ureter in the Female Pelvis

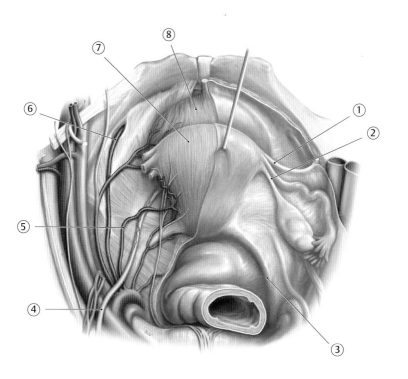

Ureter in the Female Pelvis

① round lig. of uterus
② lig. of ovary
③ rectouterine (uterosacral) fold
④ ureter
⑤ uterine a.
⑥ obturator a.
⑦ uterus
⑧ urinary bladder

❋ The ureter crosses the pelvic brim at the bifurcation of the common iliac artery and then passes under the uterine artery within the transverse cervical (cardinal) ligament as it courses forward toward the urinary bladder.

Fig. 21.7. From *Atlas of Anatomy, Third Edition*, p. 249.

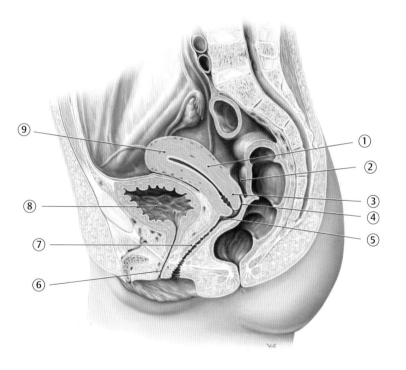

Female Pelvis, Sagittal Section

①   body of uterus

②   rectouterine pouch

③   cervix of uterus

④   posterior vaginal fornix

⑤   anterior vaginal fornix

⑥   urethra

⑦   vagina

⑧   urinary bladder

⑨   fundus of uterus

✴ The rectouterine pouch is the lowest point of the female pelvis. Fluid that may accumulate here can be accessed by needle aspiration through the posterior vaginal fornix.

Fig. 21.8A. From *Atlas of Anatomy, Third Edition*, p. 250.

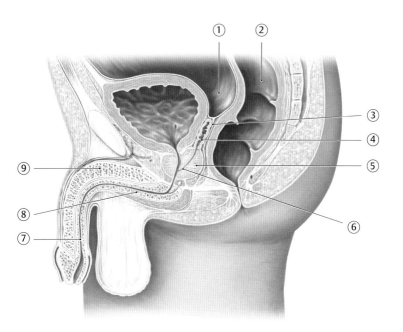

Male Pelvis, Sagittal Section

①   rectovesical pouch

②   rectum

③   rectovesical septum

④   ductus deferens, ampulla

⑤   prostate

⑥   ejaculatory duct

⑦   urethra, spongy part

⑧   penis, corpus spongiosum

⑨   penis, corpus cavernosum

❋ The right and left ejaculatory ducts form by the union of the ducts from the seminal glands and the ampullae of the ductus deferens on each side.

Fig. 21.10A. From *Atlas of Anatomy, Third Edition*, p. 251.

Urinary Bladder and Prostate

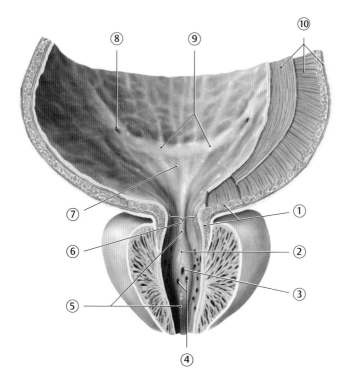

What are the boundaries of the trigone of the bladder?

Urinary Bladder and Prostate

①   internal urethral sphincter

②   seminal colliculus

③   prostatic utricle

④   openings of ejaculatory ducts

⑤   prostatic urethra

⑥   neck of bladder

⑦   trigone of bladder

⑧   ureteral orifice

⑨   interureteric crest

⑩   detrusor muscle

❗ The boundaries of the trigone are defined by lines connecting the right and left ureteral orifices and the neck of the bladder.

Fig. 21.10C. From *Atlas of Anatomy, Third Edition*, p. 251.

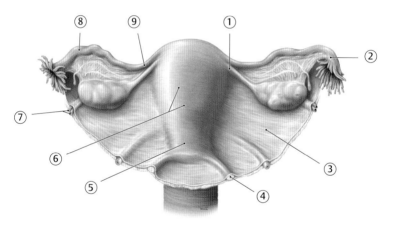

Where is the most common site of fertilization?

① lig. of ovary

② infundibulum

③ mesometrium of broad lig.

④ uterosacral lig.

⑤ cervix of uterus

⑥ body of uterus

⑦ ovarian a. and v.

⑧ ampulla of uterine tube

⑨ isthmus of uterine tube

❗ Fertilization most often occurs in the ampulla of the uterine tube.

Fig. 21.17A. From *Atlas of Anatomy, Third Edition*, p. 255.

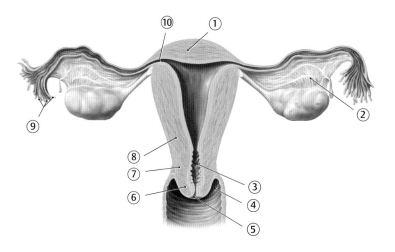

Uterus and Uterine Tube II

①   fundus of uterus

②   mesovarium

③   cervical canal

④   vaginal fornix, lateral part

⑤   external os

⑥   cervix, vaginal part

⑦   cervix, supravaginal part

⑧   myometrium

⑨   fimbriae at ostium

⑩   uterine ostium

Fig. 21.17B. From *Atlas of Anatomy, Third Edition*, p. 255.

Female External Genitalia

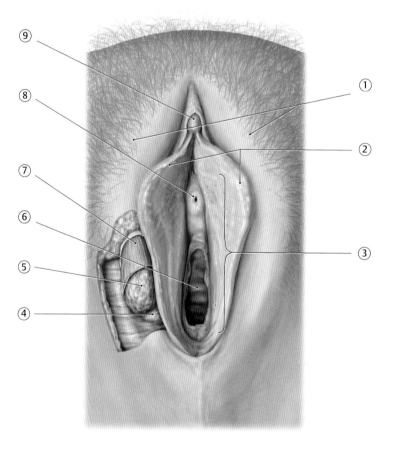

Female External Genitalia

① labia majora

② labia minora

③ vestibule of vagina

④ greater vestibular (Bartholin) gland

⑤ vestibular bulb

⑥ vaginal orifice

⑦ bulbospongiosus

⑧ external urethral orifice

⑨ glans of clitoris

Erectile Tissues in the Female

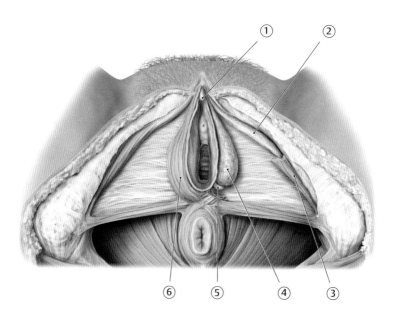

Erectile Tissues in the Female

①   glans of clitoris
②   crus of clitoris
③   ischiocavernosus
④   vestibular bulb
⑤   greater vestibular gland
⑥   bulbospongiosus

Fig. 21.27. From *Atlas of Anatomy, Third Edition*, p. 261.

Penis

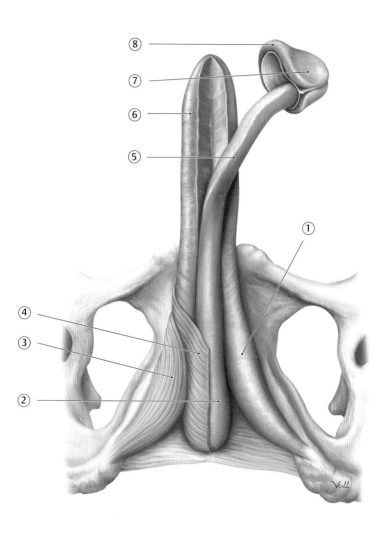

🔲 Which part(s) of the penis encloses the urethra?

Penis

1. crus of penis
2. bulb of penis
3. ischiocavernosus
4. bulbospongiosus
5. corpus spongiosum
6. corpus cavernosum
7. glans of penis
8. corona of glans

! The male urethra is enclosed within the bulb of the penis and the corpus spongiosum.

Fig. 21.28A. From *Atlas of Anatomy, Third Edition*, p. 262.

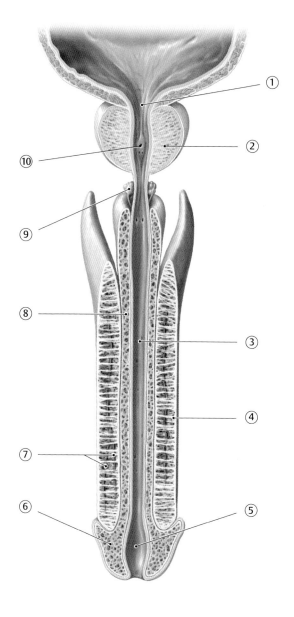

Penis, Longitudinal Section

1. urethra, preprostatic part
2. prostate
3. urethra, spongy part
4. corpus cavernosum
5. navicular fossa
6. glans of penis
7. branches of deep penile a.
8. corpus spongiosum
9. bulbourethral gland
10. seminal colliculus

Fig. 21.28B. From *Atlas of Anatomy, Third Edition*, p. 262.

Assessory Sex Glands

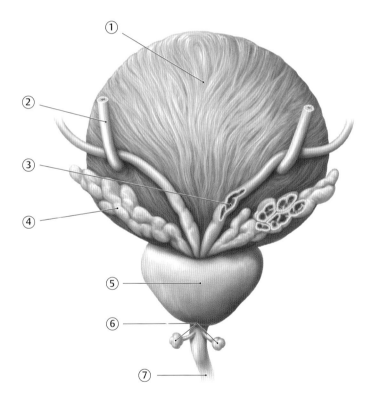

Assessory Sex Glands

1. urinary bladder
2. ureter
3. ductus deferens, ampulla
4. seminal gland
5. prostate
6. bulbourethral glands
7. urethra

Fig. 21.31. From *Atlas of Anatomy, Third Edition*, p. 264.

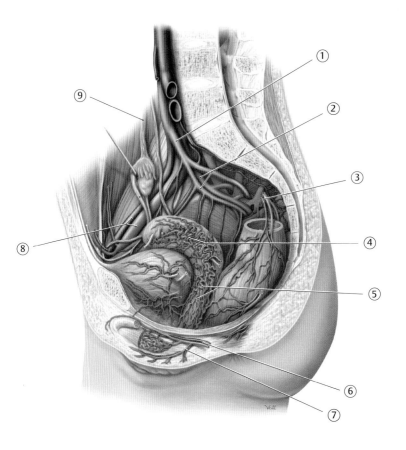

Blood Vessels of the Pelvis, Female

① right internal iliac a.

② internal iliac a. and v., anterior divisions

③ superior rectal a. and v.

④ uterine venous plexus

⑤ vaginal venous plexus

⑥ left internal pudendal a. and v.

⑦ perineal a. and v.

⑧ right external iliac a. and v.

⑨ right ovarian a. and v. (in suspensory lig.)

Fig. 22.1B. From *Atlas of Anatomy, Third Edition*, p. 267.

Blood Vessels of the Rectum

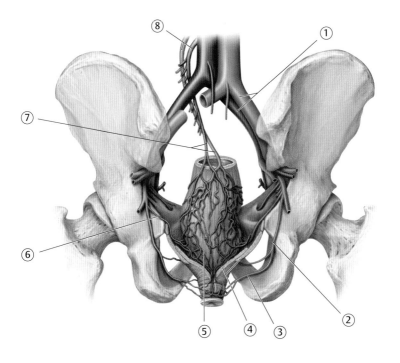

❓ The rectum is described as the site of a portocaval anastomosis. Explain what this means.

Blood Vessels of the Rectum

① right common iliac a. and v.
② right internal pudendal v.
③ right inferior rectal v.
④ levator ani
⑤ rectal venous plexus
⑥ left middle rectal a.
⑦ superior rectal a. and v.
⑧ inferior mesenteric a. and v.

! The upper rectum is drained by the superior rectal veins, which drain into the portal venous system. The inferior rectal veins drain the lower rectum into the internal and common iliac veins, which drain into the inferior vena cava (caval system). The middle rectal veins act as the connection between these two venous systems. The direction of venous flow into either system is determined by pressure within the veins.

Fig. 22.2. From *Atlas of Anatomy, Third Edition*, p. 268.

Blood Vessels of the Female Genitalia

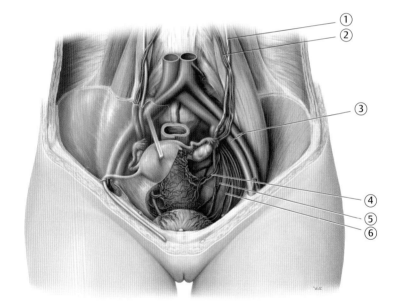

Blood Vessels of the Female Genitalia

① left ureter
② left ovarian a. and v.
③ left external iliac a. and v.
④ uterine a. and v.
⑤ vaginal a.
⑥ superior vesical a. and vesical v.

Fig. 22.4A. From *Atlas of Anatomy, Third Edition*, p. 269.

Blood Vessels of the Male Genitalia

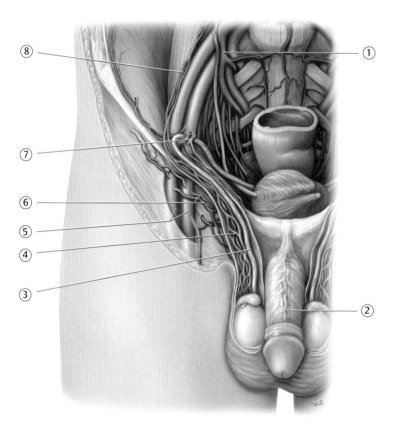

⁉ Describe the asymmetrical venous drainage of the testes.

Blood Vessels of the Male Genitalia

① internal iliac a. and v.

② dorsal penile a. , deep dorsal v.

③ right ductus deferens

④ pampiniform plexus

⑤ femoral a. and v.

⑥ external pudendal a. and v.

⑦ inferior epigastric a. and v.

⑧ testicular a. and v.

⚠ The right testicular vein drains directly into the inferior vena cava. The left testicular vein drains first to the left renal vein, which in turn drains to the inferior vena cava.

Fig. 22.4B. From *Atlas of Anatomy, Third Edition*, p. 269.

Innervation of Pelvic Viscera, Male

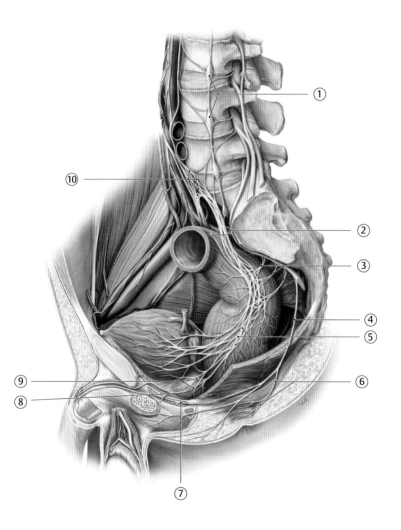

With reference to the image above, what types of nerve fibers are carried in #2, #3, and # 4?

Innervation of Pelvic Viscera, Male

①   sympathetic trunk, lumbar ganglia

②   left hypogastric n.

③   pelvic splanchnic nn.

④   pudendal n.

⑤   inferior rectal plexus

⑥   inferior rectal nn.

⑦   dorsal n. of penis

⑧   cavernous nn. of penis

⑨   prostatic plexus

⑩   superior hypogastric plexus

⚠ Hypogastric nerves (#2) carry only sympathetic fibers and pelvic splanchnic nerves (#3) carry only parasympathetic fibers. The pudendal nerve (#4) is primarily a somatic nerve, although it carries some sympathetic fibers to perineal structures.

Fig. 22.16. From *Atlas of Anatomy, Third Edition*, p. 275.

Upper Limb

(Continued)

Upper Limb

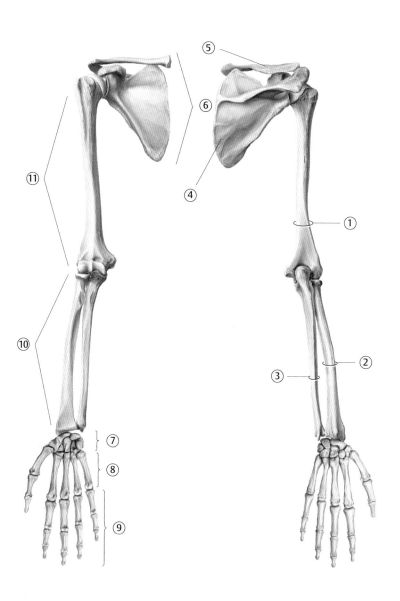

Bones of the Upper Limb

1. humerus
2. radius
3. ulna
4. scapula
5. clavicle
6. shoulder girdle
7. carpals
8. metacarpals
9. phalanges
10. forearm
11. arm

Clavicle

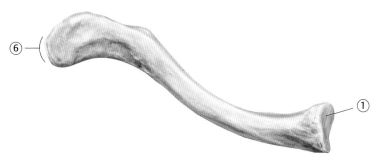

A. Superior view

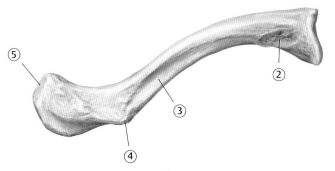

B. Inferior view

Clavicle

①   sternal articular surface

②   impression for costoclavicular lig.

③   groove for subclavius m.

④   conoid tubercle

⑤   acromial articular surface

⑥   acromial end

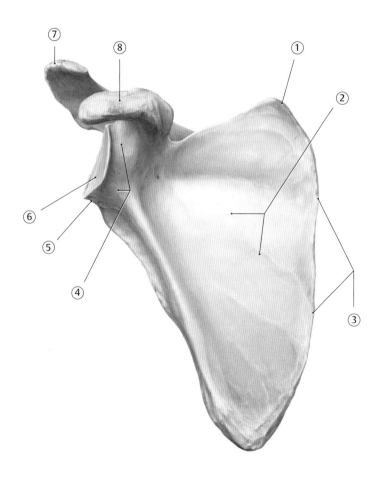

Scapula, Anterior View

① superior angle
② subscapular fossa
③ medial border
④ neck
⑤ infraglenoid tubercle
⑥ glenoid cavity
⑦ acromion
⑧ coracoid process

Fig. 25.4A. From *Atlas of Anatomy, Third Edition*, p. 295.

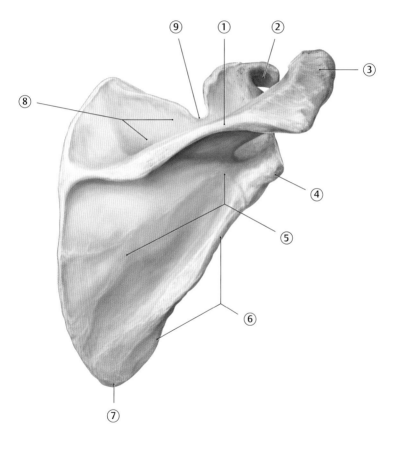

Scapula, Posterior View

1. scapular spine
2. coracoid process
3. acromion
4. infraglenoid tubercle
5. infraspinous fossa
6. lateral border
7. inferior angle
8. supraspinous fossa
9. scapular notch

Fig. 25.4C. From *Atlas of Anatomy, Third Edition*, p. 295.

Humerus

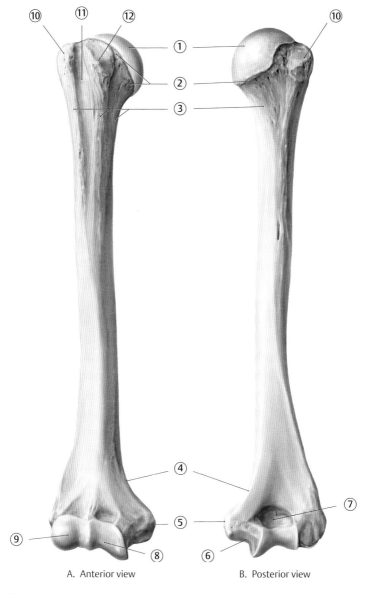

A. Anterior view   B. Posterior view

Which neurovascular structures are at risk for injury in a fracture of the humerus at the surgical neck?

Humerus

1. head of humerus
2. anatomical neck
3. surgical neck
4. medial supracondylar ridge
5. medial epicondyle
6. ulnar groove
7. olecranon fossa
8. trochlea
9. capitulum
10. greater tubercle
11. intertubercular groove
12. lesser tubercle

⚠️ The axillary n., with the anterior and posterior humeral circumflex aa., encircle the surgical neck and may be injured by a fracture in this location.

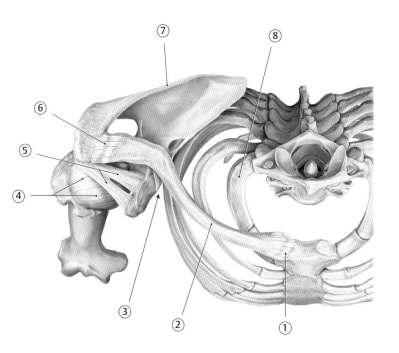

Joints of the Shoulder Girdle

① sternoclavicular joint

② clavicle

③ scapulothoracic joint

④ glenohumeral joint

⑤ coracoacromial lig.

⑥ acromioclavicular joint

⑦ scapula

⑧ 1st rib

✱ The sternoclavicular joint is the only bony articulation between the trunk and the shoulder girdle. The scapula "articulates" with the trunk only through muscular attachments. During movements of the shoulder girdle, the scapula glides on the curved surface between the serratus anterior and subscapularis in a functional relationship known as the scapulothoracic joint.

Fig. 25.7. From *Atlas of Anatomy, Third Edition*, p. 298.

Sternoclavicular Joint

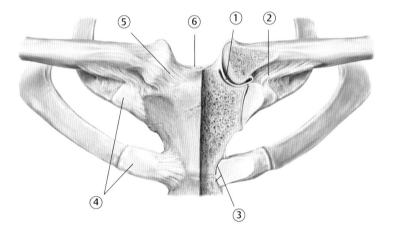

Sternoclavicular Joint

① articular disk
② costoclavicular lig.
③ sternocostal joint
④ costal cartilage
⑤ anterior sternoclavicular lig.
⑥ interclavicular lig.

✽ A fibrocartilaginous articular disk compensates for the mismatch of surfaces between the two saddle-shaped articular facets of the clavicle and manubrium sterni.

Fig. 25.9. From *Atlas of Anatomy, Third Edition*, p. 299.

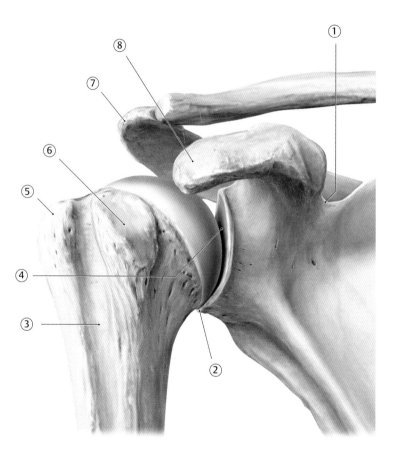

Glenohumeral Joint: Bony Elements

①   scapular notch
②   infraglenoid tubercle
③   intertubercular groove
④   glenoid cavity
⑤   greater tubercle
⑥   lesser tubercle
⑦   acromion
⑧   coracoid process

Fig. 25.11A. From *Atlas of Anatomy, Third Edition*, p. 300.

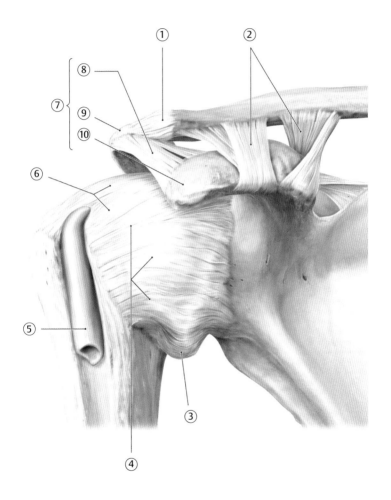

🔋 What role does the coracoacromial arch play in stabilizing the shoulder joint?

Glenohumeral Joint: Capsule and Ligaments

①   acromioclavicular lig.

②   coracoclavicular lig.

③   axillary recess

④   joint capsule, glenohumeral ligs.

⑤   intertubercular synovial sheath

⑥   coracohumeral lig.

⑦   coracoacromial arch

⑧   coracoacromial lig.

⑨   acromion

⑩   coracoid process

! The coracoacromial lig., stretching between the coracoid process and the acromion, helps prevent superior dislocation of the humerus.

Fig. 25.13. From *Atlas of Anatomy, Third Edition*, p. 301.

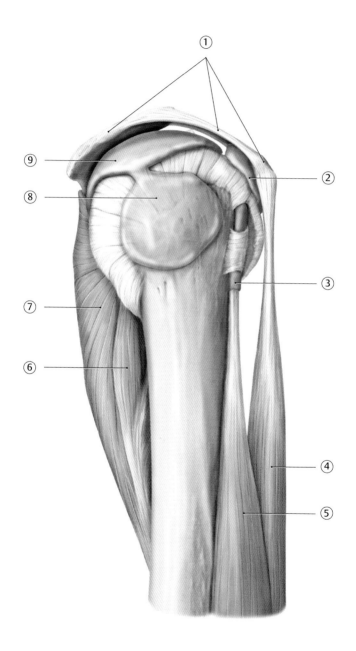

Subacromial Space

1. coracoacromial arch
2. subtendinous bursa of subscapularis
3. intertubercular tendon sheath
4. biceps brachii, short head
5. biceps brachii, long head
6. teres minor
7. infraspinatus
8. subdeltoid bursa
9. subacromial bursa

Subacromial Bursa and Glenoid Cavity

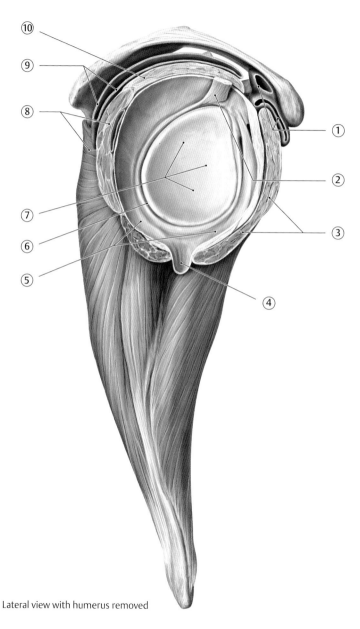

Lateral view with humerus removed

What is the function of the glenoid labrum?

Subacromial Bursa and Glenoid Cavity

① subtendinous bursa of subscapularis

② tendon of biceps brachii, long head

③ subscapularis

④ axillary recess

⑤ joint capsule

⑥ glenoid labrum

⑦ glenoid cavity

⑧ infraspinatus

⑨ subacromial bursa

⑩ supraspinatus

⚠ The glenoid labrum is a rim of fibrocartilage attached to the shallow bony glenoid cavity. It deepens the articular surface for the large humeral head.

Fig. 25.16. From *Atlas of Anatomy, Third Edition*, p. 302.

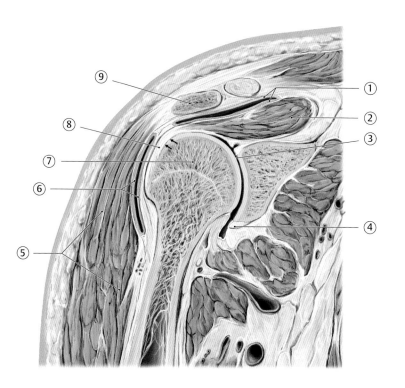

Shoulder, Coronal Section

① subacromial bursa

② supraspinatus

③ glenoid cavity

④ glenoid labrum

⑤ deltoid

⑥ subdeltoid bursa

⑦ head of humerus

⑧ supraspinatus tendon

⑨ acromion

❈ Degenerative changes and chronic inflammation of the supraspinatus tendon can cause the tendon to fray and rupture. When the subacromial and subdeltoid bursae tear in conjunction with the ruptured tendon, they become continuous with the cavity of the glenohumeral joint.

Fig. 25.17B. From *Atlas of Anatomy, Third Edition*, p. 303.

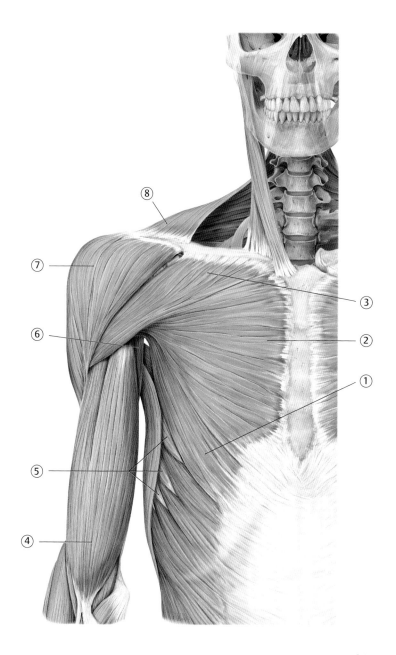

Superficial Muscles of the Anterior Shoulder and Arm: Pectoralis Major and Coracobrachialis

① pectoralis major, clavicular part

② pectoralis major, sternocostal part

③ pectoralis major, abdominal part

④ biceps brachii

⑤ serratus anterior

⑥ coracobrachialis

⑦ deltoid

⑧ trapezius

Muscle		Origin	Insertion	Innervation	Action
Pectoralis major	Clavicular part	Clavicle (medial half)	Humerus (crest of greater tubercle)	Medial and lateral pectoral nn. (C5–T1)	Entire muscle: Adduction, internal rotation Clavicular and sternocostal parts: Flexion, assist in respiration when shoulder is fixed
	Sternocostal part	Sternum and costal cartilages 1–6			
	Abdominal part	Rectus sheath (anterior layer)			
Coracobrachialis		Scapula (coracoid process)	Humerus (in line with crest of lesser tubercle)	Musculocutaneous nn. (C5–C7)	Flexion, adduction, internal rotation

Fig. 25.18A. From *Atlas of Anatomy, Third Edition*, p. 304.

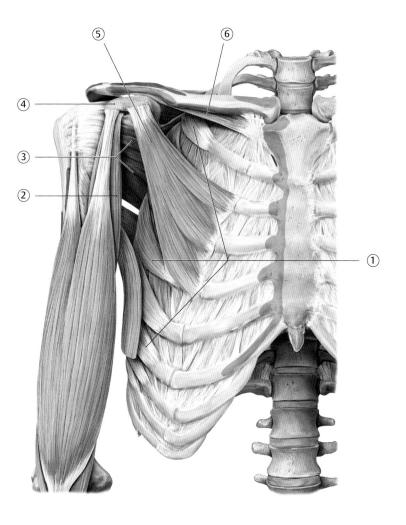

Deep Muscles of the Anterior Shoulder and Arm: Subclavius, Pectoralis Minor, and Serratus Anterior

①   serratus anterior

②   coracobrachialis

③   subscapularis

④   coracoid process

⑤   pectoralis minor

⑥   subclavius

Muscle		Origin	Insertion	Innervation	Action
Subclavius		1st rib	Clavicle (inferior surface)	Nerve to subclavius (C5, C6)	Steadies the clavicle in the sternoclavicular joint
Pectoralis minor		3rd–5th ribs	Coracoid process	Medial pectoral n. (C8, T1)	Draws scapula downward, causing inferior angle to move posteromedially; rotates glenoid inferiorly; assists in respiration
Serratus interior	Superior part	1st–9th ribs	Scapula (costal and dorsal surfaces of superior angle)	Long thoracic n. (C5–C7)	Superior part: Lowers the raised arm
	Intermediate part		Scapula (costal surface of medial border)		Entire muscle: Draws scapula laterally forward; elevates ribs when shoulder is fixed
	Inferior part		Scapula (costal surface of medial border and costal and dorsal surfaces of inferior angle)		Inferior part: Rotate inferior angle of scapula laterally forward (allows elevation of arm above 90°)

Fig. 25.18B. From *Atlas of Anatomy, Third Edition*, p. 305.

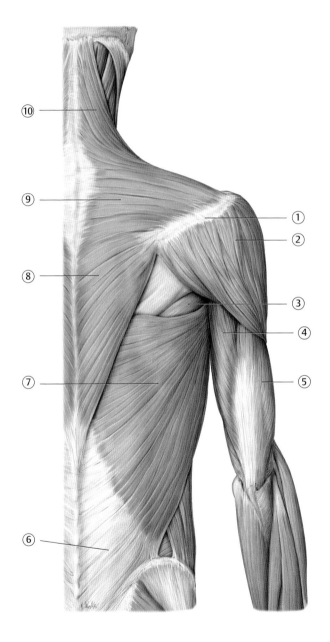

Superficial Muscles of the Posterior Shoulder and Arm: Trapezius

①   scapular spine

②   deltoid

③   teres major

④   triceps brachii, long head

⑤   triceps brachii, lateral head

⑥   thoracolumbar fascia

⑦   latissimus dorsi

⑧   trapezius, ascending part

⑨   trapezius, transverse part

⑩   trapezius, descending part

Muscle		Origin	Insertion	Innervation	Action
Trapezius	Descending part	Occipital bone; spinous processes of C1–C7	Clavicle (lateral one third)	Accessory n. (CN XI); C3–C4 of cervical plexus	Draws scapula obliquely upward; rotates glenoid cavity superiorly; tilts head to same side and rotates it to opposite
	Transverse part	Aponeurosis at T1–T4 spinous processes	Acromion		Draws scapula medially
	Ascending part	Spinous processes of T5–T12	Scapular spine		Draws scapula medially downward
					Entire muscle: Steadies scapula on thorax
CN, cranial nerve.					

Fig. 25.20A. From *Atlas of Anatomy, Third Edition*, p. 308.

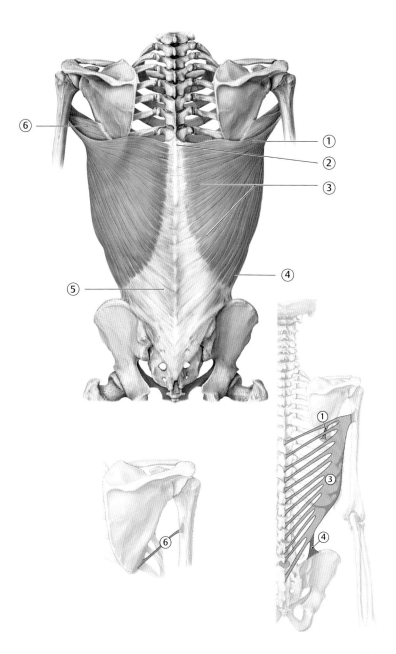

Superficial Muscles of the Posterior Shoulder and Arm: Latissimus Dorsi and Teres Major

① latissimus dorsi, scapular part

② T7 spinous process

③ latissimus dorsi, vertebral part

④ latissimus dorsi, iliac part

⑤ thoracolumbar fascia

⑥ teres major

Muscle		Origin	Insertion	Innervation	Action
Latissimus dorsi	Vertebral part	Spinous processes of T7–T12 vertebrae; thoracolumbar fascia	Floor of the intertubercular groove of the humerus	Thoracodorsal n. (C6–C8)	Internal rotation, adduction, extension, respiration ("cough muscle")
	Scapular part	Scapula (inferior angle)			
	Costal part	9th–12th ribs			
	Iliac part	Iliac crest (posterior one third)			
Teres major		Scapula (inferior angle)	Crest of lesser tubercle of the humerus (anterior angle)	Lower subscapular n. (C5–C7)	Internal rotation, adduction, extension

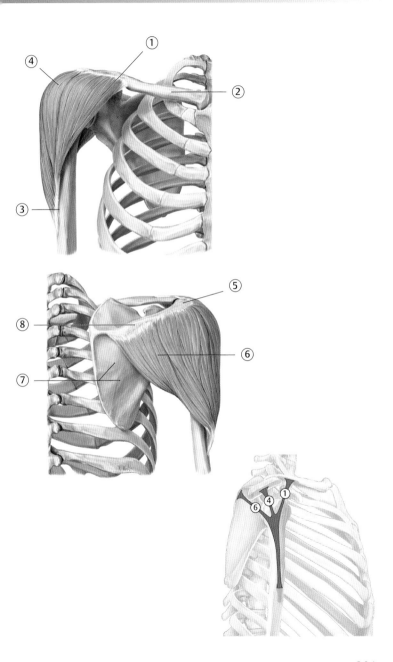

Superficial Muscles of the Posterior Shoulder and Arm: Deltoid

① deltoid, clavicular part

② clavicle

③ deltoid tuberosity

④ deltoid, acromial part

⑤ acromion

⑥ deltoid, spinal part

⑦ scapula, posterior surface

⑧ scapular spine

Muscle		Origin	Insertion	Innervation	Action*
Deltoid	Clavicular part	Lateral one third of clavicle	Humerus (deltoid tuberosity)	Axillary n. (C5, C6)	Flexion, internal rotation, adduction
	Acromial part	Acromion			Abduction
	Spinal part	Scapular spine			Extension, external rotation, adduction
*Between 60 and 90 degrees of abduction, the clavicular and spinal parts assist the acromial part with abduction.					

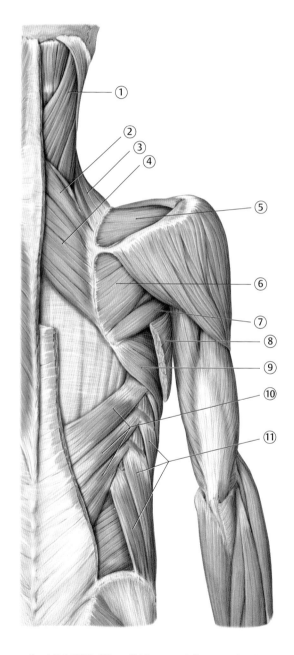

Deep Muscles of the Posterior Shoulder and Arm: Levator Scapulae, Rhomboid Major and Minor

① splenius capitis

② rhomboid minor

③ levator scapulae

④ rhomboid major

⑤ supraspinatus

⑥ infraspinatus

⑦ teres major

⑧ latissimus dorsi

⑨ serratus anterior

⑩ serratus posterior inferior

⑪ external oblique

Muscle	Origin	Insertion	Innervation	Action
Levator scapulae	Transverse processes of C1–C4	Scapula (superior angle)	Dorsal scapular n. and cervical spinal nn. (C3–C4)	Draws scapula medially upward while moving inferior angle medially; inclines neck to same side
Rhomboid minor	Spinous processes of C6, C7	Medial border of scapula above (minor) and below (major) scapular spine	Dorsal scapular n. (C4–C5)	Steadies scapula; draws scapula medially upward
Rhomboid major	Spinous processes of T1–T4 vertebrae			

Fig. 25.20B. From *Atlas of Anatomy, Third Edition*, p. 309.

Muscles of the Rotator Cuff

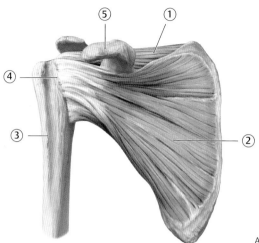

A. Anterior view

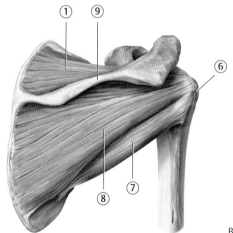

B. Posterior view

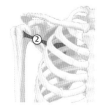

C. Anterior view

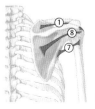

D. Posterior view

Muscles of the Rotator Cuff

①   supraspinatus

②   subscapularis

③   crest of greater tubercle

④   lesser tubercle

⑤   coracoid process

⑥   greater tubercle

⑦   teres minor

⑧   infraspinatus

⑨   scapular spine

Muscle	Origin	Insertion		Innervation	Action
Supraspinatus	Scapula	Supraspinous fossa	Humerus (greater tubercle)	Suprascapular n. (C4–C6)	Abduction
Infraspinatus		Infraspinous fossa			External rotation
Teres minor		Lateral border	Humerus	Axillary n. (C5, C6)	External rotation, weak adduction
Subscapularis		Subscapular fossa	Humerus (lesser tubercle)	Subscapular n. (C5, C6)	Internal rotation

Fig. 25.23A,B,C,D. From *Atlas of Anatomy, Third Edition*, p. 313.

Muscles of the Anterior Arm: Biceps Brachii and Brachialis

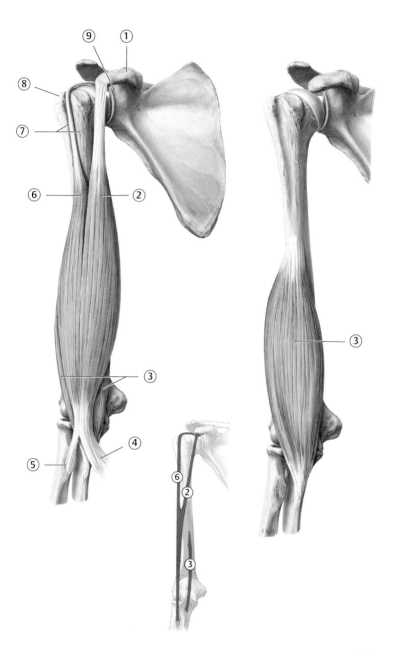

Muscles of the Anterior Arm: Biceps Brachii and Brachialis

① coracoid process

② biceps brachii, short head

③ brachialis

④ bicipital aponeurosis

⑤ radial tuberosity, biceps brachii tendon

⑥ biceps brachii, long head

⑦ intertubercular groove

⑧ greater tubercle

⑨ supraglenoid tubercle

Muscle		Origin	Insertion	Innervation	Action
Biceps brachii	Long head	Supraglenoid tubercle of scapula	Radial tuberosity and bicipital aponeurosis	Musculocutaneous n. (C5–C6)	Elbow joint: Flexion; supination* Shoulder joint: Flexion; stabilization of humeral head during deltoid contraction; abduction and internal rotation of the humerus
	Short head	Coracoid process of scapula			
Brachialis		Humerus (distal half of anterior surface)	Ulnar tuberosity	Musculocutaneous n. (C5–C6) and radial n. (C7, minor)	Flexion at the elbow joint
*When the elbow is flexed, the biceps brachii acts as a powerful supinator because the lever arm is almost perpendicular to the axis of pronation/supination.					

Muscles of the Posterior Arm: Triceps Brachii and Anconeus

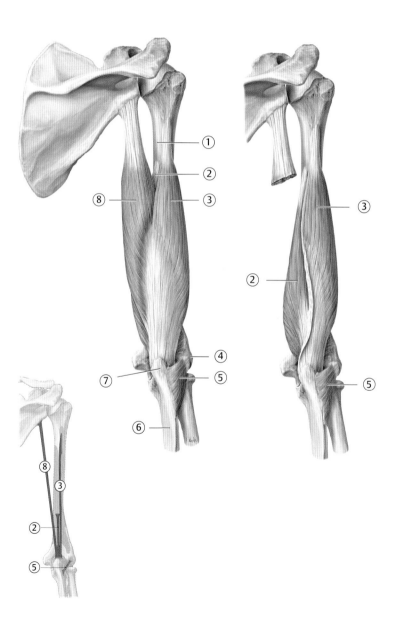

Muscles of the Posterior Arm: Triceps Brachii and Anconeus

①   shaft of humerus

②   triceps brachii, medial head

③   triceps brachii, lateral head

④   lateral epicondyle

⑤   anconeus

⑥   ulna

⑦   olecranon

⑧   triceps brachii, long head

Muscle		Origin	Insertion	Innervation	Action
Triceps brachii	Long head	Scapula (infraglenoid tubercle)	Olecranon of ulna	Radial n. (C6–C8)	Elbow joint: Extension Shoulder joint, long head: Extension and adduction
	Medial head	Posterior humerus, distal to radial groove; medial intermuscular septum			
	Lateral head	Posterior humerus, proximal to radial groove; lateral intermuscular septum			
Anconeus		Lateral epicondyle of humerus (variance: posterior joint capsule)	Olecranon of ulna (radial surface)		Extends the elbow and tightens its joint

Fig. 25.31A,C,D. From *Atlas of Anatomy, Third Edition*, p. 319.

Radius and Ulna

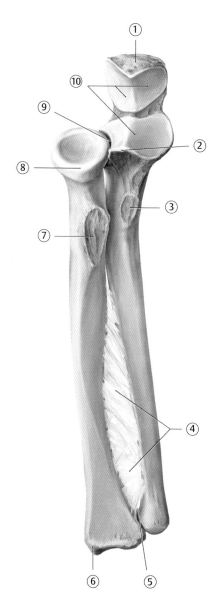

🔲 What type of movement occurs at the proximal and distal radioulnar joints?

Radius and Ulna

1. olecranon
2. coronoid process
3. ulnar tuberosity
4. interosseous membrane
5. distal radioulnar joint
6. styloid process of radius
7. radial tuberosity
8. head of radius
9. proximal radioulnar joint
10. trochlear notch

Pronation and supination occur at the proximal and distal radioulnar joints.

Fig. 26.1C. From *Atlas of Anatomy, Third Edition*, p. 321.

Ligaments of the Elbow Joint

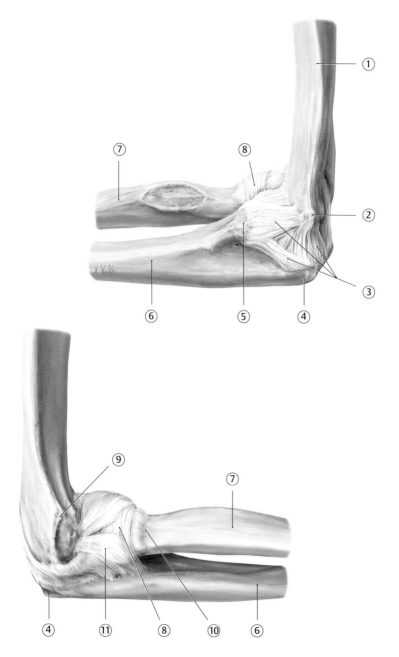

Ligaments of the Elbow Joint

① humerus
② medial epicondyle
③ ulnar collateral lig.
④ olecranon
⑤ coronoid process
⑥ ulna
⑦ radius
⑧ anular lig. of radius
⑨ lateral epicondyle
⑩ neck of radius
⑪ radial collateral lig.

Joints and ligaments of the elbow

Joint	Articulating surfaces		Ligament
Humeroulnar joint	Trochlea	Ulna (trochlear notch)	Ulnar collateral lig.
Humeroradial joint	Capitulum	Radius (articular fovea)	Radial collateral lig.
Proximal radioulnar joint	Radius (articular circumference)	Ulna (radial notch)	Anular lig. of radius

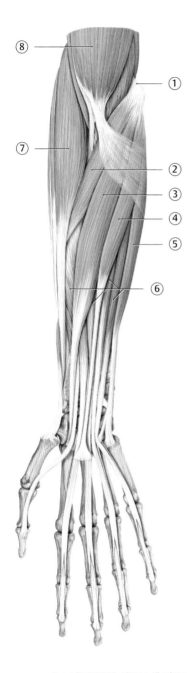

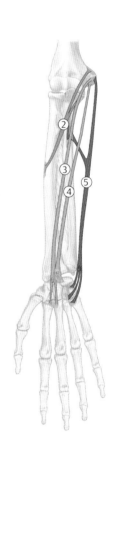

Superficial Muscles of the Anterior Forearm

① common head of flexors at medial epicondyle

② pronator teres

③ flexor carpi radialis

④ palmaris longus

⑤ flexor carpi ulnaris

⑥ flexor digitorum superficialis

⑦ brachioradialis

⑧ biceps brachii

Muscle	Origin	Insertion	Innervation	Action
Pronator teres	Humeral head: Medial epicondyle of humerus Ulnar head: Coronoid process	Lateral radius (distal to supinator insertion)	Median n. (C6, C7)	Elbow: weak flexion Forearm: pronation
Flexor carpi radialis	Medial epicondyle of humerus	Base of 2nd metacarpal (variance: base of 3rd metacarpal)		Wrist: flexion and abduction (radial deviation) of hand
Palmaris longus		Palmar aponeurosis	Median n. (C7, C8)	Elbow: weak flexion Wrist: flexion tightens palmar aponeurosis
Flexor carpi ulnaris	Humeral head: Medial epicondyle Ulnar head: Olecranon	Pisiform; hook of hamate; base of 5th metacarpal	Ulnar n. (C7–T1)	Wrist: flexion and adduction (ulnar deviation) of hand

Fig. 26.12A, Fig. 26.10A. From *Atlas of Anatomy, Third Edition*, pp. 332, 328.

Intermediate Muscles of the Anterior Forearm

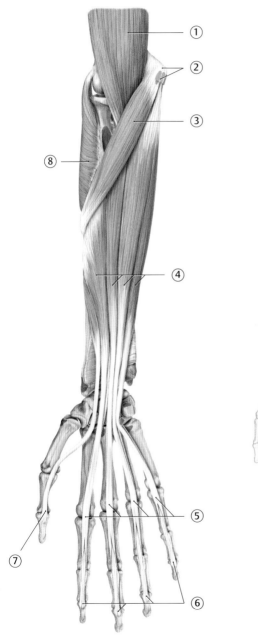

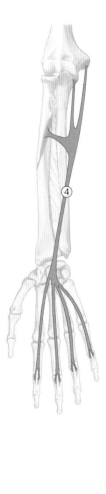

Intermediate Muscles of the Anterior Forearm

① brachialis
② medial epicondyle
③ pronator teres
④ flexor digitorum superficialis
⑤ flexor digitorum superficialis tendons
⑥ flexor digitorum profundus tendons
⑦ flexor pollicis longus
⑧ supinator

Muscle	Origin	Insertion	Innervation	Action
Flexor digitorum superficialis	Humeral-ulnar head: Medial epicondyle of humerus and coronoid process of ulna Radial head: Upper half of anterior border of radius	Sides of middle phalanges of 2nd–5th digits	Median n. (C8, T1)	Elbow: Weak flexion Wrist, MCP, and PIP joints of 2nd–5th digits: Flexion
MCP, metacarpophalangeal; PIP, proximal interphalangeal.				

Fig. 26.12B, Fig. 26.10B. From *Atlas of Anatomy, Third Edition*, pp. 332, 328.

Deep Muscles of the Anterior Forearm

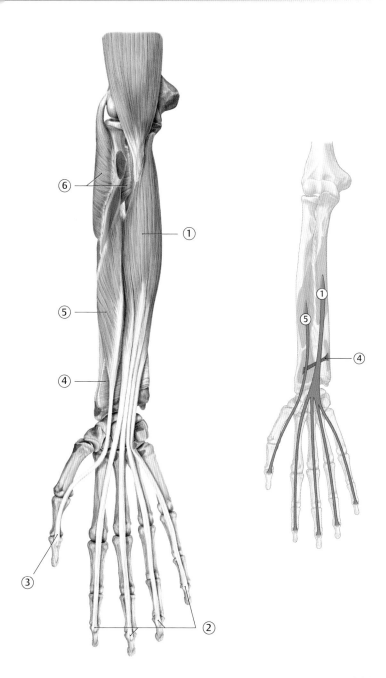

Deep Muscles of the Anterior Forearm

1. flexor digitorum profundus
2. flexor digitorum profundus tendons
3. flexor pollicis longus tendon
4. pronator quadratus
5. flexor pollicis longus
6. supinator

Muscle	Origin	Insertion	Innervation	Action
Flexor digitorum profundus	Ulna (proximal two thirds of flexor surface) and interosseous membrane	Distal phalanges of 2nd–5th digits (palmar surface)	Median n. (C8, T1, radial half of fingers 2 and 3) Ulnar n. (C8, T1, ulnar half of fingers 4 and 5)	Wrist, MCP, PIP, and DIP joints of 2nd–5th digits: Flexion
Flexor pollicis longus	Radius (midanterior surface) and adjacent interosseous membrane	Distal phalanx of thumb (palmar surface)	Median n. (C8, T1)	Wrist: Flexion and abduction (radial deviation) of hand Carpometacarpal joint of thumb: Flexion MCP and IP joints of thumb: Flexion
Pronator quadratus	Distal quarter of ulna (anterior surface)	Distal quarter of radius (anterior surface)		Hand: Pronation Distal radioulnar joint: Stabilization
DIP, distal interphalangeal; IP, interphalangeal; MCP, metacarpophalangeal; PIP, proximal interphalangeal.				

Radialis Muscles of the Posterior Forearm

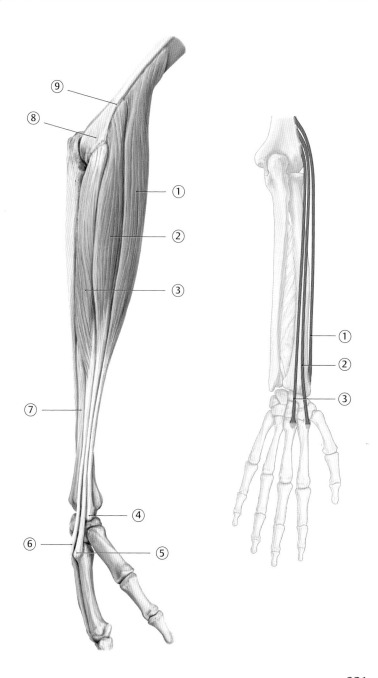

Radialis Muscles of the Posterior Forearm

① brachioradialis

② extensor carpi radialis longus

③ extensor carpi radialis brevis

④ styloid process of radius

⑤ base of 2nd metacarpal

⑥ base of 3rd metacarpal

⑦ radius

⑧ lateral epicondyle

⑨ lateral supracondylar crest

Muscle	Origin	Insertion	Innervation	Action
Brachioradialis	Distal humerus (lateral surface), lateral intermuscular septum	Styloid process of the radius	Radial n. (C5, C6)	Elbow: Flexion Forearm: Semipronation
Extensor carpi radialis longus	Lateral supracondylar ridge of distal humerus, lateral intermuscular septum	2nd metacarpal (base)	Radial n. (C6, C7)	Elbow: Weak flexion Wrist: Extension and abduction
Extensor carpi radialis brevis	Lateral epicondyle of humerus	3rd metacarpal (base)	Radial n. (C7, C8)	

Fig. 26.15, Fig. 26.16A. From *Atlas of Anatomy, Third Edition*, pp. 334, 335.

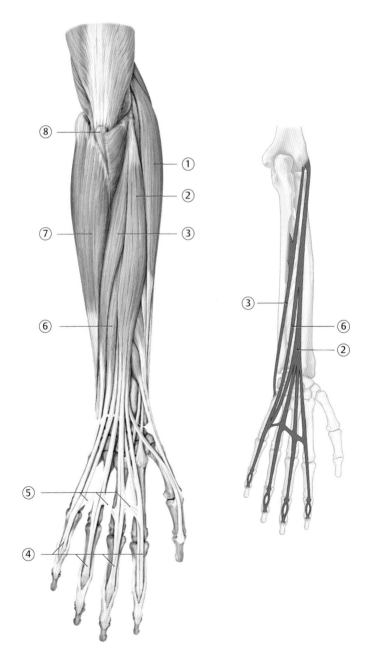

Superficial Muscles of the Posterior Forearm

① extensor carpi radialis longus

② extensor digitorum

③ extensor carpi ulnaris

④ extensor digitorum tendons, dorsal digital expansion

⑤ intertendinous connections

⑥ extensor digiti minimi

⑦ flexor carpi ulnaris

⑧ olecranon

Muscle	Origin	Insertion	Innervation	Action
Extensor digitorum	Common head (lateral epicondyle of humerus)	Dorsal digital expansion of 2nd–5th digits	Radial n. (C7, C8)	Wrist: Extension MCP, PIP, and DIP joints of 2nd–5th digits: Extension/abduction of fingers
Extensor digiti minimi		Dorsal digital expansion of 5th digit		Wrist: Extension, ulnar abduction of hand MCP, PIP, and DIP joints of 5th digit: Extension and abduction of 5th digit
Extensor carpi ulnaris	Common head (lateral epicondyle of humerus) Ulnar head (dorsal surface)	Base of 5th metacarpal		Wrist: Extension, adduction (ulnar deviation) of hand

DIP, distal interphalangeal; MCP, metacarpophalangeal; PIP, proximal interphalangeal.

Fig. 26.17, Fig. 26.11A. From *Atlas of Anatomy, Third Edition*, pp. 336, 330.

Deep Muscles of the Posterior Forearm

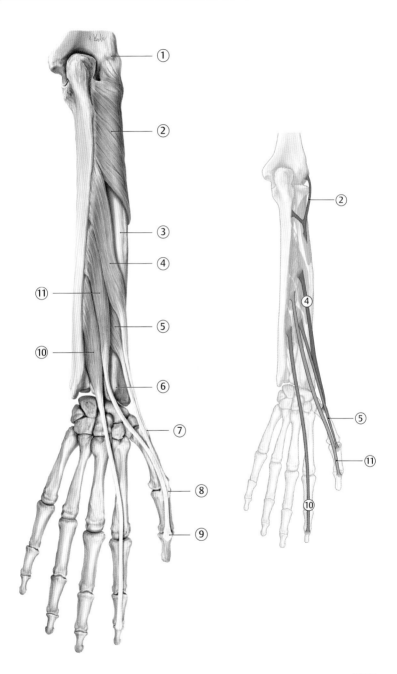

Deep Muscles of the Posterior Forearm

① lateral epicondyle
② supinator
③ radius
④ abductor pollicis longus
⑤ extensor pollicis brevis
⑥ dorsal tubercle
⑦ base of 1st\ metacarpal
⑧ base of 1st proximal phalanx
⑨ base of 1st distal phalanx
⑩ extensor indicis
⑪ extensor pollicis longus

Muscle	Origin	Insertion	Innervation	Action
Supinator	Olecranon, lateral epicondyle of humerus, radial collateral lig., annular lig. of radius	Radius (between radial tuberosity and insertion of pronator teres)	Radial n. (C6, C7)	Radioulnar joints: Supination
Abductor pollicis longus	Radius and ulna (dorsal surfaces, interosseous membrane)	Base of 1st metacarpal	Radial n. (C7, C8)	Radiocarpal joint: Abduction of the hand Carpometacarpal joint of thumb: Abduction
Extensor pollicis brevis	Radius (posterior surface) and interosseous membrane	Base of proximal phalanx of thumb		Radiocarpal joint: Abduction (radial deviation) of hand Carpometacarpal and MCP joints of thumb: Extension
Extensor pollicis longus	Ulna (posterior surface) and interosseous membrane	Base of distal phalanx of thumb		Wrist: Extension and abduction (radial deviation) of hand Carpometacarpal joint of thumb: Adduction MCP and IP joints of thumb: Extension
Extensor indicis	Ulna (posterior surface) and interosseous membrane	Posterior digital extension of 2nd digit		Wrist: Extension MCP, PIP, and DIP joints of 2nd digit: Extension

DIP, distal interphalangeal; IP, interphalangeal; MCP, metacarpophalangeal; PIP, proximal interphalangeal.

Fig. 26.18, Fig. 26.19B. From *Atlas of Anatomy, Third Edition*, p. 336, 337.

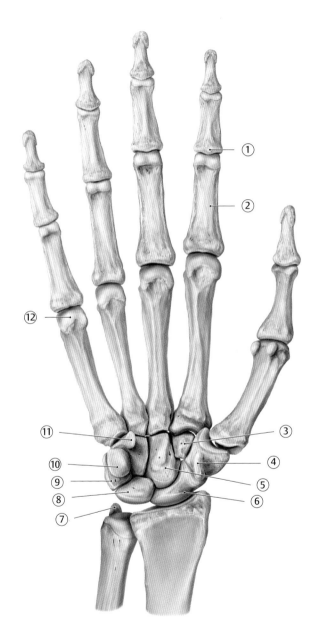

Which of the carpal bones is most frequently fractured?

Bones of the Wrist and Hand, Palmar View

1. base of 2nd middle phalanx
2. shaft of 2nd proximal phalanx
3. trapezoid
4. tubercle of trapezium
5. capitate
6. scaphoid
7. styloid process of ulna
8. lunate
9. triquetrum
10. pisiform
11. hook of hamate
12. head of 5th metacarpal

⚠ Scaphoid fractures are the most common carpal bone fractures. A fracture at its narrow waist can compromise its blood supply and result in non-union and avascular necrosis of the bone.

Fig. 27.2. From *Atlas of Anatomy, Third Edition*, p. 339.

Joints of the Wrist and Hand

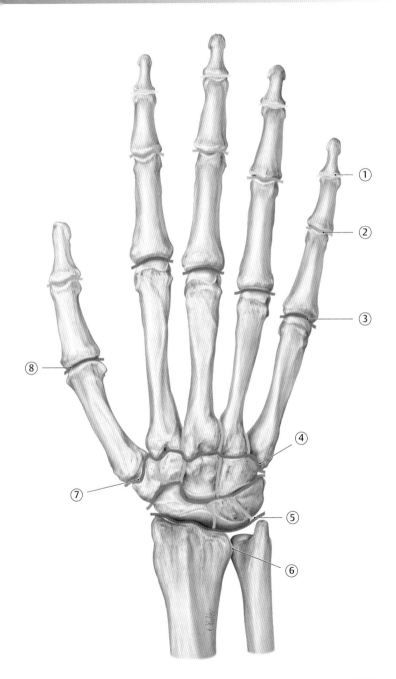

Joints of the Wrist and Hand

① distal interphalangeal joint
② proximal interphalangeal joint
③ metacarpophalangeal joint
④ carpometacarpal joints
⑤ radiocarpal joint
⑥ distal radioulnar joint
⑦ carpometacarpal joint of thumb
⑧ metacarpophalangeal joint of thumb

✱ The distal radius articulates with the scaphoid and lunate at the radiocarpal joint. The ulna articulates with the radius but is separated from the carpal bones by an articular disk.

Fig. 27.5A. From *Atlas of Anatomy, Third Edition*, p. 342.

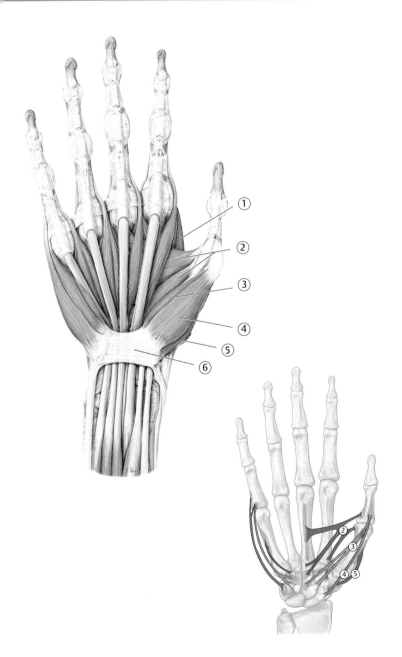

Intrinsic Muscles of the Hand: Superficial Layer—Thenar Muscles

①   1st dorsal interosseous

②   adductor pollicis, transverse and oblique heads

③   flexor pollicis brevis

④   abductor pollicis brevis

⑤   opponens pollicis

⑥   flexor retinaculum

Muscle	Origin	Insertion		Innervation		Action
Adductor pollicis	Transverse head: 3rd metacarpal (palmar surface)	Thumb (base of proximal phalanx) via the ulnar sesamoid	Via the ulnar sesamoid	Ulnar n. (C8, T1)		CMC joint of thumb: Adduction
	Oblique head: Capitate bone, 2nd and 3rd metacarpals (bases)					MCP joint of thumb: Flexion
Abductor pollicis brevis	Scaphoid bone and trapezium, flexor retinaculum	Thumb (base of proximal phalanx) via the radial sesamoid	Via the radial sesamoid	Median n. (C8, T1)	C8, T1	CMC joint of thumb: Abduction
Flexor pollicis brevis	Superficial head: Flexor retinaculum			Superficial head: Median n. (C8, T1)		CMC joint of thumb: Flexion
	Deep head: Capitate bone, trapezium			Deep head: Ulnar n. (C8, T1)		
Opponens pollicis	Trapezium	1st metacarpal (radial border)		Median n. (C8, T1)		CMC joint of thumb: Opposition
CMC, carpometacarpal; MCP, metacarpophalangeal.						

Fig. 27.18C, Fig. 27.24. From *Atlas of Anatomy, Third Edition*, pp. 351, 356.

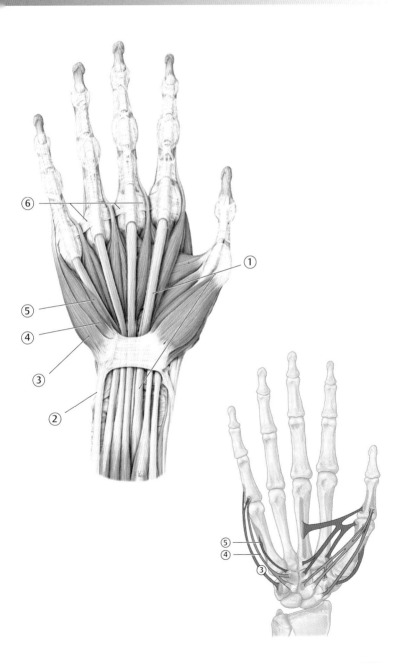

Intrinsic Muscles of the Hand: Superficial Layer—Hypothenar Muscles

① flexor digitorum superficialis tendon
② flexor carpi ulnaris tendon
③ abductor digiti minimi
④ flexor digiti minimi brevis
⑤ opponens digiti minimi
⑥ deep transverse metacarpal lig.

Muscle	Origin	Insertion	Innervation	Action
Opponens digiti minimi	Hook of hamate, flexor retinaculum	5th metacarpal (ulnar border)	Ulnar n. (C8, T1)	Draws metacarpal in palmar direction (opposition)
Flexor digiti minimi brevis		5th proximal phalanx (base)		MCP joint of little finger: Flexion
Abductor digiti minimi	Pisiform bone	5th proximal phalanx (ulnar base) and dorsal digital expansion of 5th digit		MCP joint of little finger: Flexion and abduction of little finger PIP and DIP joints of little finger: Extension
Palmaris brevis	Palmar aponeurosis (ulnar border)	Skin of hypothenar eminence		Tightens the palmar aponeurosis (protective function)

DIP, distal interphalangeal; MCP, metacarpophalangeal; PIP, proximal interphalangeal.

Fig. 27.18C, Fig. 27.24. From *Atlas of Anatomy, Third Edition*, pp. 351, 356.

Intrinsic Muscles of the Hand: Middle Layer—Lumbricals

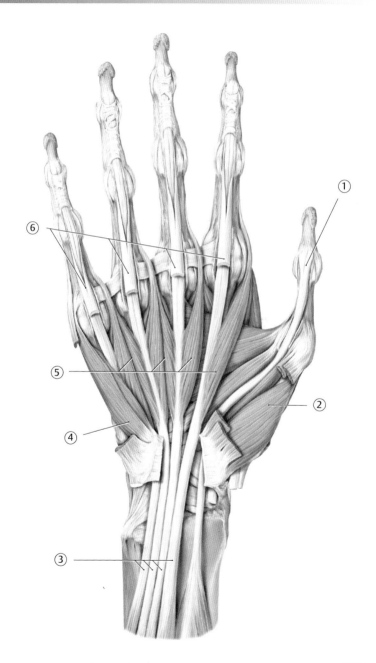

Intrinsic Muscles of the Hand: Middle Layer—Lumbricals

① flexor pollicis longus tendon

② opponens pollicis

③ flexor digitorum profundus tendons

④ flexor digiti minimi brevis

⑤ 1st–4th lumbricals

⑥ flexor digitorum superficialis tendons

Muscle group	Muscle	Origin	Insertion	Innervation	Action
Lumbricals	1st	Tendons of flexor digitorum profundus (radial sides)	2nd digit (dde)	Median n. (C8, T1)	2nd–5th digits: • MCP joints: Flexion • Proximal and distal IP joints: Extension
	2nd		3rd digit (dde)		
	3rd	Tendons of flexor digitorum profundus (bipennate from medial and lateral sides)	4th digit (dde)	Ulnar n. (C8, T1)	
	4th		5th digit (dde)		

dde, dorsal digital expansion; IP, interphalangeal; MCP, metacarpophalangeal.

Fig. 27.18D. From *Atlas of Anatomy, Third Edition*, p. 351.

Intrinsic Muscles of the Hand: Middle and Deep Layers

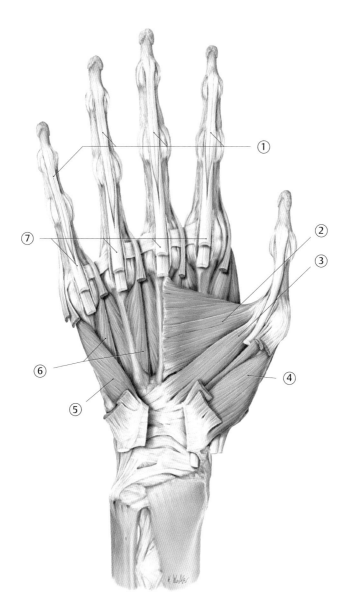

What is the innervation of the lumbricals and interossei?

Intrinsic Muscles of the Hand: Middle and Deep Layers

① flexor digitorum profundus tendons
② adductor pollicis, transverse head
③ adductor pollicis, oblique head
④ opponens pollicis
⑤ opponens digiti minimi
⑥ 2nd and 3rd palmar interossei
⑦ flexor digitorum superficialis tendons

⚠ The ulnar n. innervates most of the intrinsic muscles of the palm, including the palmar and dorsal interossei, and the 3rd and 4th lumbricals. The 1st and 2nd lumbricals are innervated by the median n.

Fig. 27.19A. From *Atlas of Anatomy, Third Edition*, p. 352.

Intrinsic Muscles of the Hand: Deep Layer—Interossei

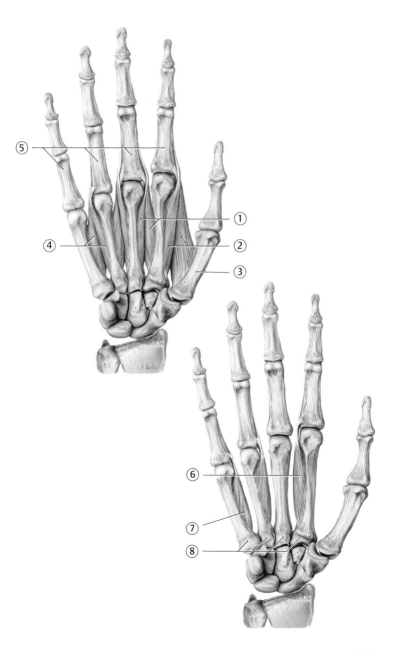

Intrinsic Muscles of the Hand: Deep Layer—Interossei

① 2nd dorsal interosseous
② 1st dorsal interosseous
③ 1st metacarpal
④ 4th dorsal interosseous
⑤ 2nd–5th proximal phalanges
⑥ 1st palmar interosseous
⑦ 3rd palmar interosseous
⑧ 2nd–5th metacarpals

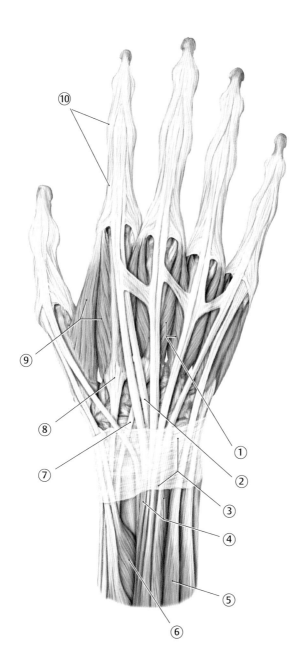

Muscles and Tendons on the Dorsum of the Hand

①   3rd dorsal interosseus

②   extensor indicis tendon

③   extensor retinaculum

④   extensor digitorum

⑤   extensor digiti minimi

⑥   extensor pollicis brevis

⑦   extensor carpi radialis brevis tendon

⑧   extensor carpi radialis longus tendon

⑨   1st dorsal interosseous

⑩   dorsal digital expansion

❂ The dorsal digital expansion (dorsal hood) allows the long digital extensors and the short muscles of the palm to act on all three finger joints.

Fig. 27.22. From *Atlas of Anatomy, Third Edition*, p. 354.

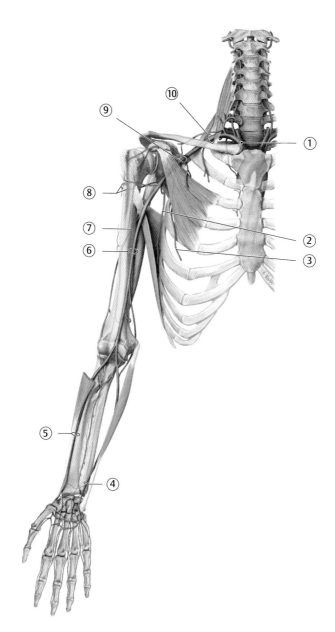

Trace the course of the major arteries of the upper limb.

Arteries of the Upper Limb

① brachiocephalic trunk
② thoracodorsal a.
③ lateral thoracic a.
④ ulnar a.
⑤ radial a.
⑥ brachial a.
⑦ deep a. of the arm
⑧ anterior and posterior circumflex humeral aa.
⑨ thoracoacromial a.
⑩ subclavian a.

! Subclavian aa. arise from the brachiocephalic trunk on the right and the aortic arch on the left. They course through the root of the neck and enter the axilla as they pass over the 1st rib. Here they become the axillary aa. At the inferior edge of the teres major, they enter the arm and are called brachial aa. These bifurcate in the cubital fossa into ulnar and radial aa., which terminate in the hand as the superficial and deep palmar arches.

Fig. 28.1B. From *Atlas of Anatomy, Third Edition*, p. 360.

Superficial Veins of the Upper Limb

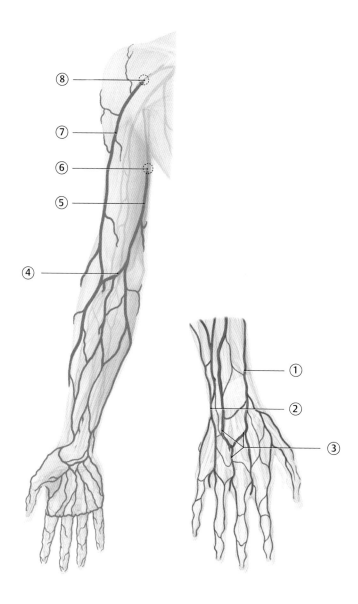

Into which deep veins do the cephalic and basilic vv. drain?

Superficial Veins of the Upper Limb

① cephalic v.
② basilic v.
③ dorsal venous network
④ median cubital
⑤ basilic v.
⑥ basilic hiatus
⑦ cephalic v.
⑧ deltopectoral groove

! The cephalic v. travels in the deltopectoral groove before it drains into the axillary v., just medial to the pectoralis minor. The basilic v. pierces the brachial fascia in the arm at the basilic hiatus, where it joins the deep brachial vv. to form the axillary v.

Nerves of the Upper Limb

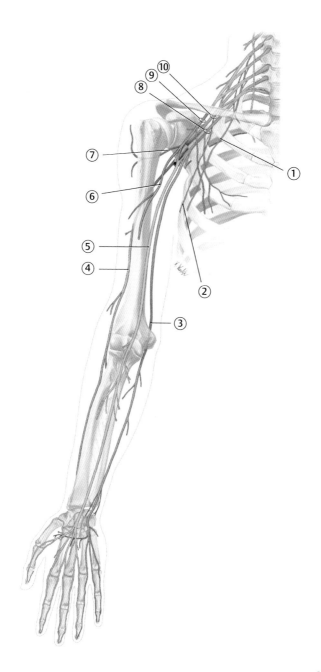

Nerves of the Upper Limb

① long thoracic n.

② thoracodorsal n.

③ ulnar n.

④ radial n.

⑤ median n.

⑥ musculocutaneous n.

⑦ axillary n.

⑧ medial cord

⑨ lateral cord

⑩ posterior cord

Nerves of the Brachial Plexus

Supraclavicular part			
Direct branches from the anterior rami or plexus trunks			
Dorsal scapular n.			C4–C5
Suprascapular n.			C4–C6
Nerve to the subclavius			C5–C6
Long thoracic n.			C5–C7
Infraclavicular part			
Short and long branches from the plexus cords			
Lateral cord	Lateral pectoral n.		C5–C7
	Musculocutaneous n.		C6–C7
	Median n.	Lateral root	
		Medial root	
Medial cord	Medial pectoral n.		C8–T1
	Medial antebrachial cutaneous n.		
	Medial brachial cutaneous n.		T1
	Ulnar n.		C7–T1
Posterior cord	Upper subscapular n.		C5–C6
	Thoracodorsal n.		C6–C8
	Lower subscapular n.		C5–C6
	Axillary n.		
	Radial n.		C5–T1

Table 28.1. From *Atlas of Anatomy, Third Edition*, p. 364.

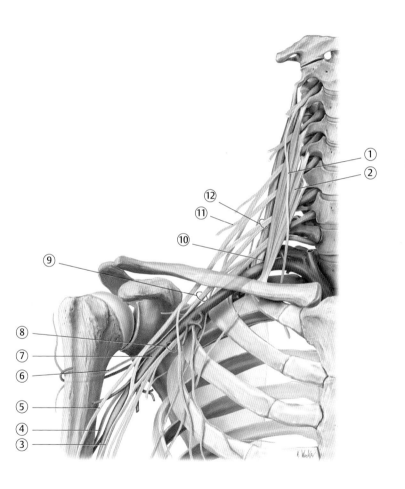

Which spinal nerves contribute to the brachial plexus?

Brachial Plexus

① phrenic n.

② anterior scalene

③ median n.

④ radial n.

⑤ musculocutaneous n.

⑥ axillary n.

⑦ axillary a.

⑧ medial cord

⑨ posterior cord

⑩ interscalene space

⑪ suprascapular n.

⑫ middle trunk

❗ The brachial plexus arises from the anterior rami of spinal nerves C5–T1

Fig. 28.11. From *Atlas of Anatomy, Third Edition*, p. 365.

Triangular and Quadrangular Spaces

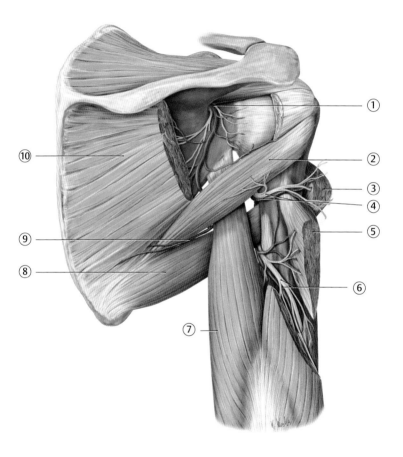

🔲 Which major vessels form the anastomosis known as the scapular arcade?

Triangular and Quadrangular Spaces

① suprascapular a. and n. in scapular notch

② teres minor

③ deltoid

④ axillary n. and posterior circumflex humeral a. in quadrangular space

⑤ triceps brachii, lateral head

⑥ deep a. of arm and radial n. in radial groove

⑦ triceps brachii, long head

⑧ teres major

⑨ circumflex scapular a. in triangular space

⑩ infraspinatus

! The suprascapular and transverse cervical (via its dorsal scapular branch) aa. of the thyrocervical trunk anastomose with the subscapular branch of the axillary a. to form this arcade.

Fig. 28.30B. From *Atlas of Anatomy, Third Edition*, p. 377.

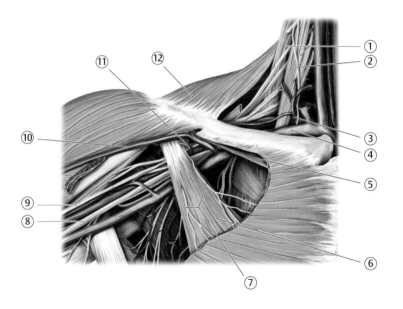

Axilla, Deep Dissection

① scalene mm.
② phrenic n.
③ thyrocervical trunk
④ subclavian v.
⑤ subclavius
⑥ pectoralis minor
⑦ medial and lateral pectoral nn.
⑧ ulnar n.
⑨ median n.
⑩ cephalic v.
⑪ thoracoacromial a.
⑫ trapezius

Fig. 28.33. From *Atlas of Anatomy, Third Edition*, p. 379.

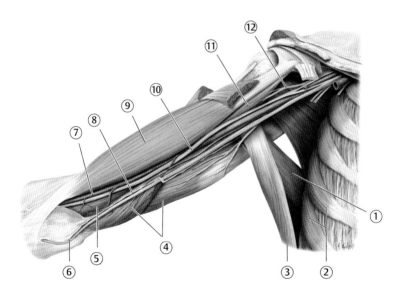

Brachial Region

1. teres major
2. serratus anterior
3. latissimus dorsi
4. triceps brachii, medial and long heads
5. brachialis
6. ulnar n.
7. brachial a.
8. medial intermuscular septum
9. biceps brachii
10. median n.
11. coracobrachialis
12. musculocutaneous n.

Fig. 28.35. From *Atlas of Anatomy, Third Edition*, p. 382.

Anterior Forearm, Deep Dissection

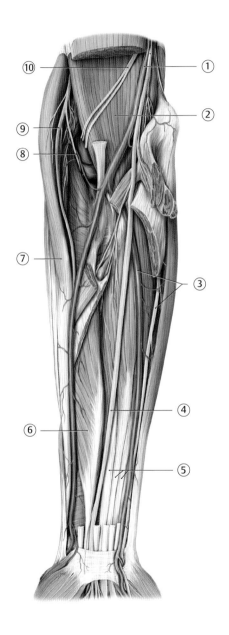

❓ Which muscles of the forearm are innervated by the ulnar n.?

Anterior Forearm, Deep Dissection

① brachial a.

② brachialis

③ ulnar a. and n.

④ median n.

⑤ flexor digitorum profundus tendons

⑥ flexor pollicis longus

⑦ brachioradialis

⑧ deep branch of radial n.

⑨ superficial branch of radial n.

⑩ musculocutaneous n.

⚠ The ulnar n. innervates the flexor carpi ulnaris and the medial half of the flexor digitorum profundus, which is associated with the 3rd and 4th digits. Most muscles of the anterior forearm are innervated by the median n.

Fig. 28.37C. From *Atlas of Anatomy, Third Edition*, p. 385.

Ulnar and Carpal Tunnels

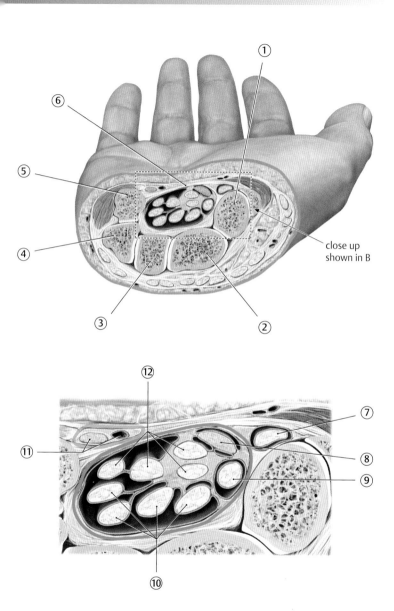

close up shown in B

What are the boundaries of the carpal and ulnar tunnels?

Ulnar and Carpal Tunnels

① scaphoid
② capitate
③ hamate
④ triquetrum
⑤ pisiform
⑥ flexor retinaculum
⑦ flexor carpi radialis tendon
⑧ median n.
⑨ flexor pollicis longus tendon
⑩ flexor digitorum profundus tendons
⑪ ulnar a. and n.
⑫ flexor digitorum superficialis tendons

! The carpal tunnel, through which the flexor tendons and median n. pass into the palm, is bounded by the flexor retinaculum and the carpal bones. The ulnar tunnel, a passage for the ulnar a. and n., is bounded by the flexor retinaculum and the palmar carpal lig.

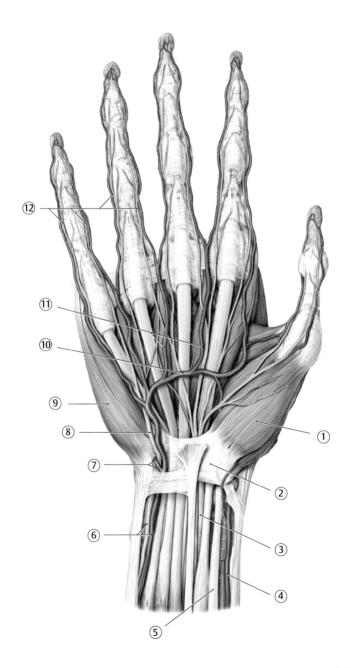

Deep Neurovascular Structures of the Palm

① abductor pollicis brevis
② flexor retinaculum
③ median n.
④ radial a.
⑤ flexor carpi radialis
⑥ ulnar a. and n.
⑦ ulnar a. and n. deep branches
⑧ ulnar n. superficial branch
⑨ abductor digiti minimi
⑩ superficial palmar arch
⑪ common palmar digital aa.
⑫ palmar digital nn.

Fig. 28.44A. From *Atlas of Anatomy, Third Edition*, p. 389.

Anatomic Snuffbox

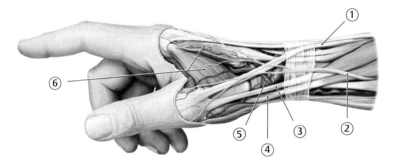

Which carpal bone lies in the floor of the anatomical snuffbox?

Anatomic Snuffbox

①   extensor pollicis longus

②   radial n., superficial branch

③   extensor pollicis brevis tendon

④   abductor pollicis longus tendon

⑤   radial a.

⑥   1st dorsal interosseous

⚠ The snuffbox is an area on the radial side of the wrist bounded by the tendons of the extensor pollicis longus, extensor pollicis brevis, and abductor pollicis longus. Because the scaphoid forms most of its floor, pain or deep tenderness in this area is associated with fractures of this bone.

Fig. 28.47. From *Atlas of Anatomy, Third Edition*, p. 390.

Lower Limb

(Continued)

Lower Limb

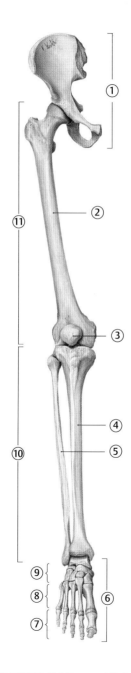

Bones of the Lower Limb

① pelvic girdle
② femur
③ patella
④ tibia
⑤ fibula
⑥ foot
⑦ phalanges
⑧ metatarsals
⑨ tarsals
⑩ lower leg
⑪ thigh

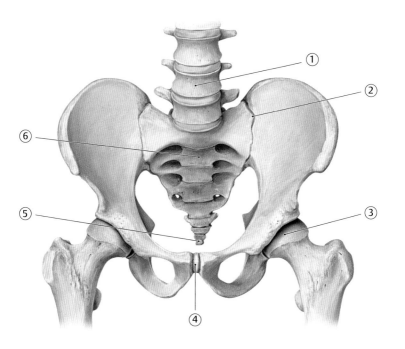

The Bony Pelvis

1. L4 vertebra
2. sacroiliac joint
3. hip joint
4. pubic symphysis
5. coccyx
6. sacrum

Fig. 31.3A. From *Atlas of Anatomy, Third Edition*, p. 405.

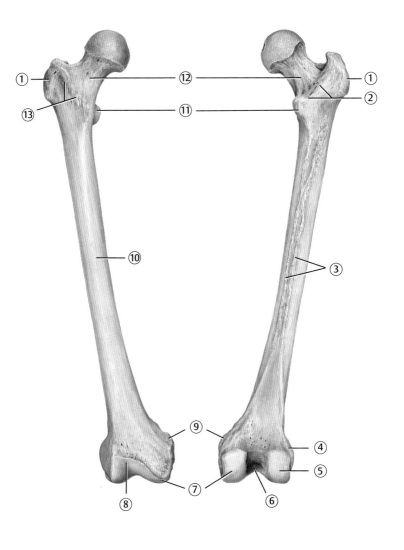

Femur

1. greater trochanter
2. intertrochanteric crest
3. linea aspera
4. lateral epicondyle
5. lateral condyle
6. intercondylar notch
7. medial condyle
8. patellar surface
9. medial epicondyle
10. shaft
11. lesser trochanter
12. neck
13. intertrochanteric line

Hip Joint: Bony Elements

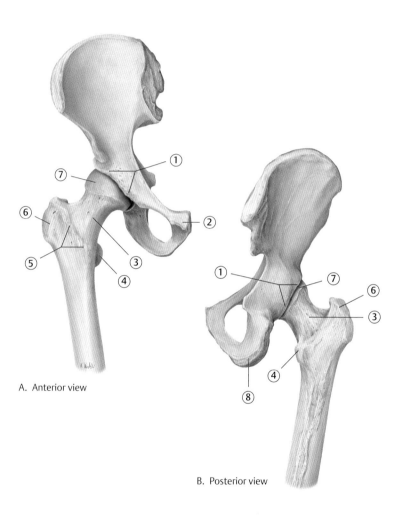

A. Anterior view

B. Posterior view

❓ How do the articulating surfaces of the hip bone and femur enhance the stability of the hip joint?

Hip Joint: Bony Elements

① acetabular rim
② pubic tubercle
③ neck of femur
④ lesser trochanter
⑤ intertrochanteric line
⑥ greater trochanter
⑦ head of femur
⑧ ischial tuberosity

❗ The head of the femur articulates with the acetabulum in a spherical, or ball-and-socket, joint. The large spherical femoral head is largely contained within the deep acetabular fossa, in contrast to the head of the humerus in the shoulder joint, which articulates with the relatively flat surface of the glenoid cavity.

Hip Joint: Capsule and Ligaments

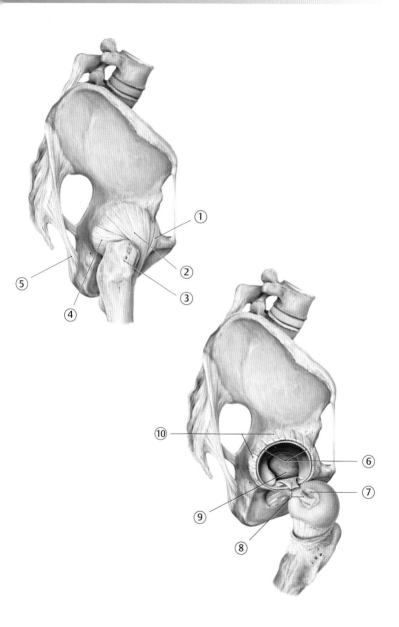

In what position is the hip joint least stable and most vulnerable to dislocation?

Hip Joint: Capsule and Ligaments

① pubofemoral lig.

② iliofemoral lig.

③ greater trochanter

④ ischiofemoral lig.

⑤ sacrotuberous lig.

⑥ acetabular labrum

⑦ fovea on femoral head

⑧ lig. of head of femur

⑨ acetabular fossa

⑩ joint capsule

⚠ The capsule of the hip joint is reinforced by three ligaments that spiral around the neck of the femur: the iliofemoral, pubofemoral, and ischiofemoral. The joint is least stable, and therefore most vulnerable to dislocation, when these ligaments are relaxed with the hip in the flexed and externally rotated position.

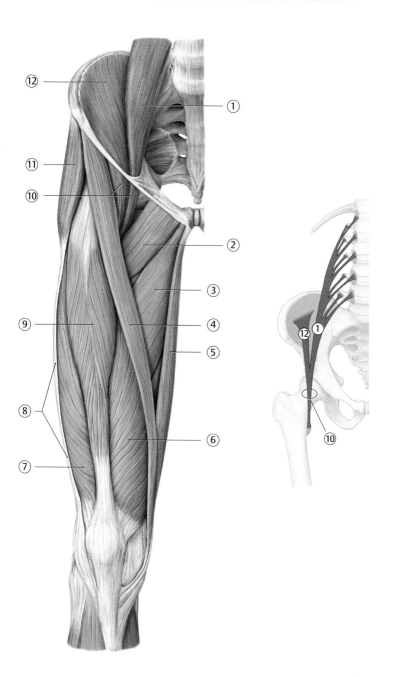

Muscles of the Anterior Hip and Thigh: Iliopsoas

① psoas major

② pectineus

③ adductor longus

④ sartorius

⑤ gracilis

⑥ vastus medialis

⑦ vastus lateralis

⑧ iliotibial tract

⑨ rectus femoris

⑩ iliopsoas

⑪ tensor fasciae latae

⑫ iliacus

Muscle		Origin	Insertion	Innervation	Action
Iliopsoas	Psoas major	*Superficial:* T12–L4 and associated intervertebral disks (lateral surfaces) *Deep:* L1–L5 vertebrae (costal processes)	Femur (lesser trochanter)	Lumbar plexus L1, L2(L3)	• Hip joint: Flexion and external rotation • Lumbar spine: *Unilateral* contraction (with the femur fixed) bends the trunk laterally to the same side *Bilateral* contraction raises the trunk from the supine position
	Iliacus	Iliac fossa		Femoral n. (L2–L3)	

Fig. 31.11A, Fig. 31.17A. From *Atlas of Anatomy, Third Edition,* pp. 412, 420.

Muscles of the Anterior Thigh: Sartorius and Quadriceps Femoris

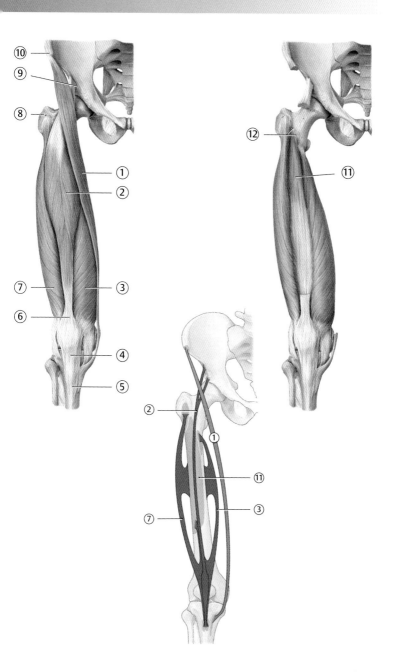

Muscles of the Anterior Thigh: Sartorius and Quadriceps Femoris

① sartorius
② rectus femoris
③ vastus medialis
④ patellar lig.
⑤ tibial tuberosity
⑥ quadriceps femoris tendon
⑦ vastus lateralis
⑧ greater trochanter
⑨ anterior inferior iliac spine
⑩ anterior superior iliac spine
⑪ vastus intermedius
⑫ intertrochanteric line

Muscle		Origin	Insertion	Innervation	Action
Sartorius		Anterior superior iliac spine	Medial to the tibial tuberosity (together with gracilis and semitendinosus)	Femoral n. (L2, L3)	• Hip joint: Flexion, abduction, and external rotation • Knee joint: flexion and internal rotation
Quadriceps femoris*	Rectus femoris	Anterior inferior iliac spine, acetabular roof of hip joint	Tibial tuberosity (via patellar lig.)	Femoral n. (L2–L4)	• Hip joint: Flexion • Knee joint: Extension
	Vastus medialis	Linea aspera (medial lip), intertrochanteric line (distal part)	Both sides of tibial tuberosity on the medial and lateral condyles (via the medial and lateral patellar retinacula)		Knee joint: Extension
	Vastus lateralis	Linea aspera (lateral lip), greater trochanter (lateral surface)			
	Vastus intermedius	Femoral shaft (anterior side)	Tibial tuberosity (via patellar lig.)		
	Articularis genus (distal fibers of vastus intermedius)	Anterior side of femoral shaft at level of the suprapatellar recess	Suprapatellar recess of knee joint capsule		Knee joint: Extension; prevents entrapment of capsule

*The entire muscle inserts on the tibial tuberosity via the patellar lig.

Fig. 31.23A,B,C. From *Atlas of Anatomy, Third Edition*, p. 424.

Muscles of the Medial Thigh: Superficial Layer

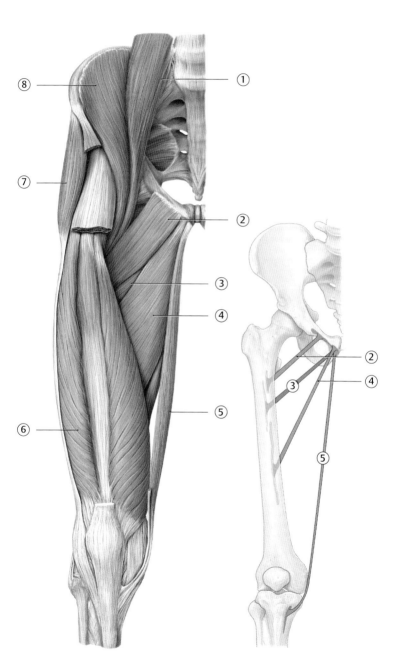

Muscles of the Medial Thigh: Superficial Layer

① psoas major

② pectineus

③ adductor brevis

④ adductor longus

⑤ gracilis

⑥ vastus lateralis

⑦ tensor fascia latae

⑧ iliacus

Muscle	Origin	Insertion	Innervation	Action
Pectineus	Pecten pubis	Femur (pectineal line and the proximal linea aspera)	Femoral n., obturator n. (L2, L3)	• Hip joint: Adduction, external rotation, and slight flexion • Stabilizes the pelvis in the coronal and sagittal planes
Adductor longus	Superior pubic ramus and anterior side of the pubic symphysis	Femur (linea aspera, medial lip in the middle third of the femur)	Obturator n. (L2–L4)	• Hip joint: Adduction and flexion (up to 70°s); extension (past 80° of flexion) • Stabilizes the pelvis in the coronal and sagittal planes
Adductor brevis	Inferior pubic ramus			
Gracilis	Inferior pubic ramus below the pubic symphysis	Tibia (medial border of the tuberosity, along with the tendons of sartorius and semitendinosus)	Obturator n. (L2, L3)	• Hip joint: Adduction and flexion • Knee joint: Flexion and internal rotation

Fig. 31.11B, Fig. 31.21A. From *Atlas of Anatomy, Third Edition*, pp. 412, 422.

Muscles of the Medial Thigh: Deep Layer

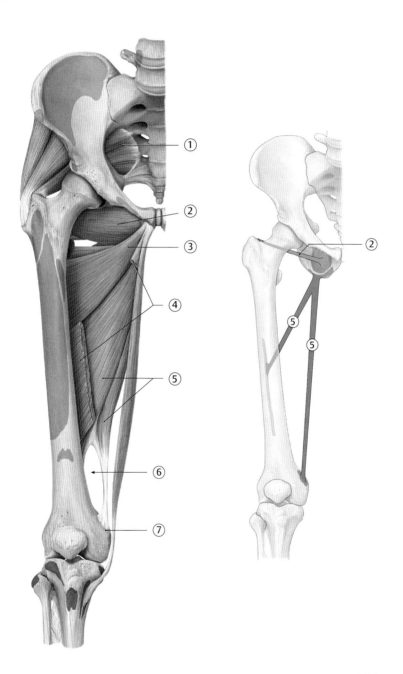

Muscles of the Medial Thigh: Deep Layer

①   piriformis

②   obturator externus

③   adductor brevis

④   adductor longus

⑤   adductor magnus

⑥   adductor hiatus

⑦   adductor tubercle

Muscle	Origin	Insertion	Innervation	Action
Obturator externus	Outer surface of the obturator membrane and its bony boundaries	Trochanteric fossa of the femur	Obturator n. (L3, L4)	• Hip joint: Adduction and external rotation • Stabilizes the pelvis in the sagittal plane
Adductor magnus	Inferior pubic ramus, ischial ramus, and ischial tuberosity	• Deep part (fleshy insertion): Medial lip of the linea aspera • Superficial part (tendinous insertion): Adductor tubercle of the femur	• Deep part: Obturator n. (L2–L4) • Superficial part: Tibial n. (L4)	• Hip joint: Adduction, extension, and slight flexion (the tendinous insertion is also active in internal rotation) • Stabilizes the pelvis in the coronal and sagittal planes

Fig. 31.11D, Fig. 31.22A. From *Atlas of Anatomy, Third Edition*, pp. 413, 423.

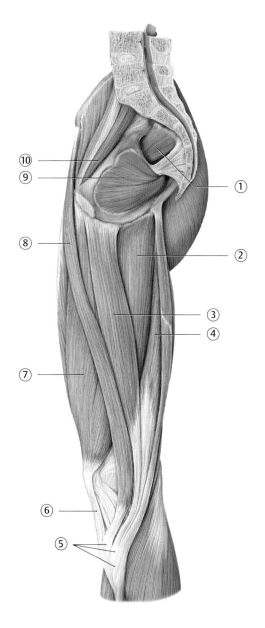

Which muscles form the pes anserinus and what are their innervations?

Medial Muscles of the Hip, Thigh, and Gluteal Region

① piriformis

② adductor magnus

③ gracilis

④ semimembranosus

⑤ pes anserinus (common tendon of insertion)

⑥ patellar lig.

⑦ vastus medialis

⑧ sartorius

⑨ obturator internus

⑩ psoas major

The pes anserinus is formed by the sartorius, innervated by the femoral n.; the gracilis, innervated by the obturator n.; and the semitendinosus, innervated by the tibial n.

Fig. 31.13. From *Atlas of Anatomy, Third Edition*, p. 415.

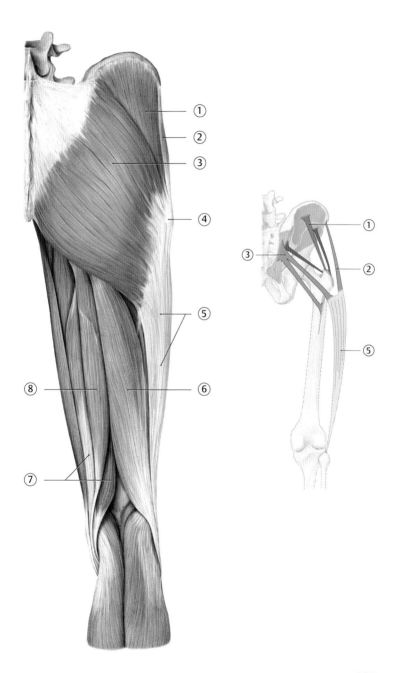

Superficial Muscles of the Gluteal Region

①   gluteus medius

②   tensor fasciae latae

③   gluteus maximus

④   greater trochanter

⑤   iliotibial tract

⑥   biceps femoris, long head

⑦   semimembranosus

⑧   semitendinosus

Muscle	Origin	Insertion	Innervation	Action
Gluteus maximus	Sacrum (dorsal surface, lateral part), ilium (gluteal surface, posterior part), thoracolumbar fascia, sacrotuberous lig.	• Upper fibers: Iliotibial tract • Lower fibers: Gluteal tuberosity	Inferior gluteal n. (L5–S2)	• Entire muscle: Extends and externally rotates the hip in sagittal and coronal planes • Upper fibers: Abduction • Lower fibers: Adduction
Gluteus medius	Ilium (gluteal surface below the iliac crest between the anterior and the posterior gluteal line)	Greater trochanter of the femur (lateral surface)	Superior gluteal n. (L4–S1)	• Entire muscle: Abducts the hip, stabilizes the pelvis in the coronal plane • Anterior part: Flexion and internal rotation • Posterior part: Extension and external rotation

Fig. 31.14A, Fig. 31.17B. From *Atlas of Anatomy, Third Edition*, pp. 416, 420.

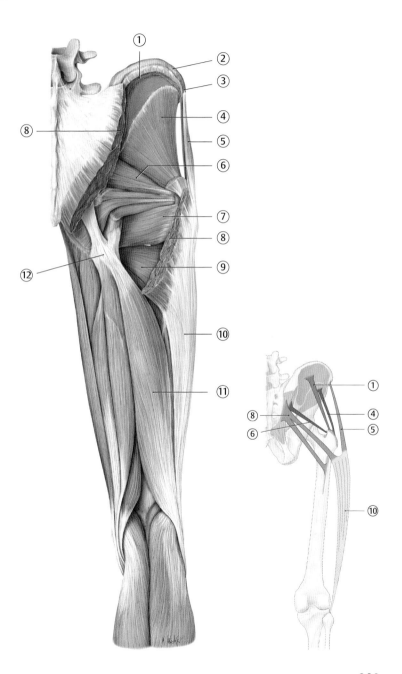

Deep Muscles of the Gluteal Region I

① gluteus medius

② iliac crest

③ anterior superior iliac spine

④ gluteus minimus

⑤ tensor fasciae latae

⑥ piriformis

⑦ quadratus femoris

⑧ gluteus maximus

⑨ adductor magnus

⑩ iliotibial tract

⑪ biceps femoris, long head

⑫ ischial tuberosity

Muscle	Origin	Insertion	Innervation	Action
Gluteus minimus	Ilium (gluteal surface below the origin of gluteus medius)	Greater trochanter of the femur (anterolateral surface)	Superior gluteal n. (L4–S1)	• Entire muscle: Abducts the hip; stabilizes the pelvis in the coronal plane • Anterior part: Flexion and internal rotation • Posterior part: Extension and external rotation
Tensor fasciae latae	Anterior superior iliac spine	Iliotibial tract		• Tenses the fascia lata • Hip joint: Abduction, flexion, and internal rotation
Piriformis	Pelvic surface of the sacrum	Apex of the greater trochanter of the femur	Sacral plexus (S1, S2)	• External rotation, abduction, and extension of the hip joint • Stabilizes the hip joint

Deep Muscles of the Gluteal Region II

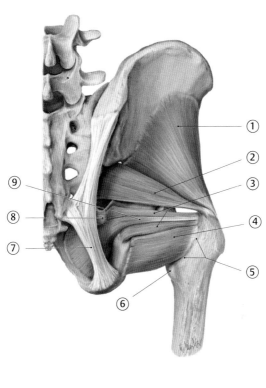

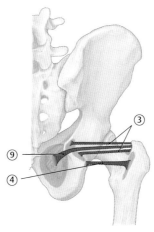

Deep Muscles of the Gluteal Region II

① gluteus minimus

② piriformis

③ gemellus superior and inferior

④ quadratus femoris

⑤ intertrochanteric crest

⑥ lesser trochanter

⑦ sacrotuberous lig.

⑧ ischial spine

⑨ obturator internus

Muscle	Origin	Insertion	Innervation	Action
Obturator internus	Inner surface of the obturator membrane and its bony boundaries	Medial surface of the greater trochanter	Sacral plexus (L5, S1)	External rotation, adduction, and extension of the hip joint (also active in abduction, depending on the joint's position)
Gemelli	• Gemellus superior: ischial spine • Gemellus inferior: ischial tuberosity	Jointly with obturator internus tendon (medial surface, greater trochanter)		
Quadratus femoris	Lateral border of the ischial tuberosity	Intertrochanteric crest of the femur		External rotation and adduction of the hip joint

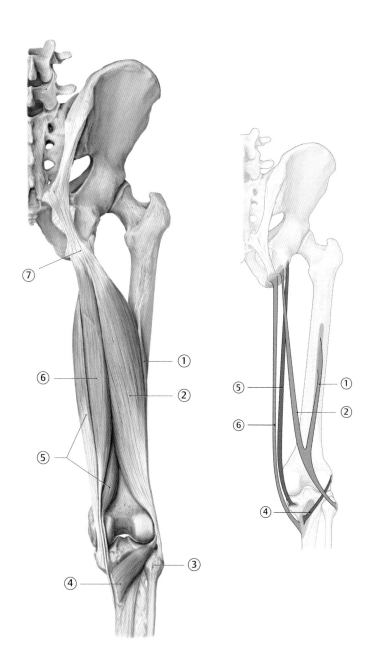

Muscles of the Posterior Thigh

① biceps femoris, short head
② biceps femoris, long head
③ fibula, head
④ popliteus
⑤ semimembranosus
⑥ semitendinosus
⑦ ischial tuberosity

Muscle	Origin	Insertion	Innervation	Action
Biceps femoris	Long head: Ischial tuberosity, sacrotuberous lig. (common head with semitendinosus)	Head of fibula	Tibial n. (L5–S2)	• Hip joint (long head): Extends the hip, stabilizes the pelvis in the sagittal plane • Knee joint: Flexion and external rotation
	Short head: Lateral lip of the linea aspera in the middle third of the femur		Common fibular n. (L5–S2)	Knee joint: Flexion and external rotation
Semimembranosus	Ischial tuberosity	Medial tibial condyle, oblique popliteal lig., popliteus fascia	Tibial n. (L5–S2)	• Hip joint: Extends the hip, stabilizes the pelvis in the sagittal plane • Knee joint: Flexion and internal rotation
Semitendinosus	Ischial tuberosity and sacrotuberous lig. (common head with long head of biceps femoris)	Medial to the tibial tuberosity in the pes anserinus (along with the tendons of gracilis and sartorius)		

Fig. 31.24A,B. From *Atlas of Anatomy, Third Edition*, p. 425.

Lateral Muscles of the Hip, Thigh, and Gluteal Region

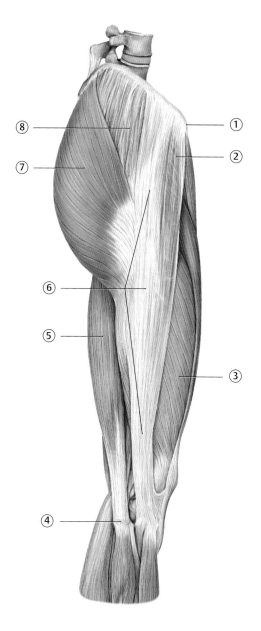

What is the iliotibial tract?

Lateral Muscles of the Hip, Thigh, and Gluteal Region

① anterior superior iliac spine

② tensor fasciae latae

③ vastus lateralis

④ fibula, head

⑤ biceps femoris, long head

⑥ iliotibial tract

⑦ gluteus maximus

⑧ gluteus medius

! The iliotibial tract is a thickened part of the fasciae latae of the thigh, reinforced by longitudinal fibers that extend from the iliac crest to the anterolateral tibia below the knee. The lateral intermuscular septum of the thigh arises from its deep surface. It encloses the tensor of the fascia lata and serves as an insertion for the aponeurosis of the gluteus maximus.

Fig. 31.16. From *Atlas of Anatomy, Third Edition*, p. 419.

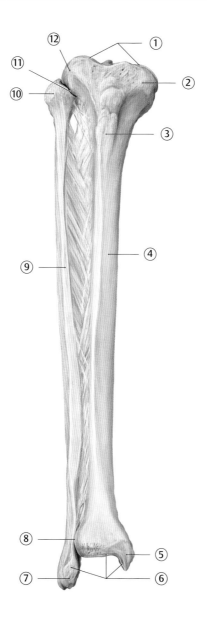

🔲 What is the role of the fibula in weight bearing and stability of the ankle?

Tibia and Fibula

① tibial plateau
② medial condyle
③ tibial tuberosity
④ tibia, shaft
⑤ medial malleolus
⑥ ankle mortise
⑦ lateral malleolus
⑧ tibiofibular syndesmosis
⑨ fibula, shaft
⑩ head of fibula
⑪ tibiofibular joint
⑫ lateral condyle

❗ The fibula has no role in weight bearing but is important in maintaining ankle stability as part of the ankle mortise. Its position is stabilized by its proximal and distal articulations with the tibia as well as the interosseous membrane. It also serves as an attachment site for several muscles of the leg.

Fig. 32.1A. From *Atlas of Anatomy, Third Edition*, p. 426.

Knee Joint: Bony Elements, Anterior View

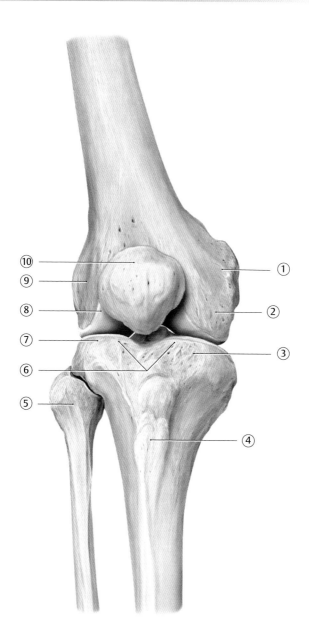

① ②
③ ④
⑤
⑥
⑦
⑧
⑨
⑩

Which bones of the lower limb articulate at the knee joint?

Knee Joint: Bony Elements, Anterior View

① medial epicondyle
② medial femoral condyle
③ medial tibial condyle
④ tibial tuberosity
⑤ head of fibula
⑥ tibial plateau
⑦ lateral tibial condyle
⑧ lateral femoral condyle
⑨ lateral epicondyle
⑩ patella

⚠ Three bones are involved in the knee joint: the femur, tibia, and patella. The fibula does not participate in the knee joint but articulates with the tibia at the proximal and distal tibiofibular joints.

Fig. 32.2A. From *Atlas of Anatomy, Third Edition*, p. 428.

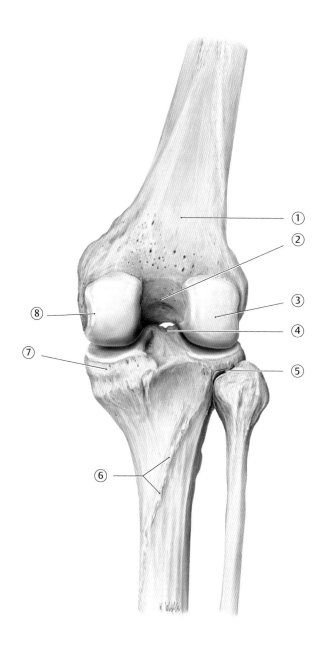

Knee Joint: Bony Elements, Posterior View

① popliteal surface
② intercondylar notch
③ lateral femoral condyle
④ intercondylar eminence
⑤ tibiofibular joint
⑥ soleal line
⑦ medial tibial condyle
⑧ medial femoral condyle

Fig. 32.2B. From *Atlas of Anatomy, Third Edition*, p. 428.

Knee Joint: Collateral and Patellar Ligaments

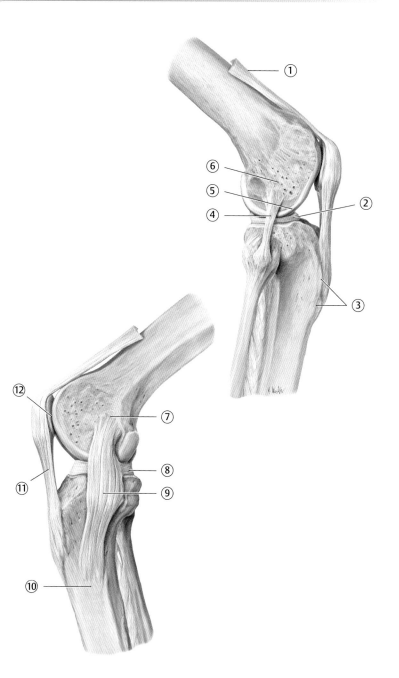

Knee Joint: Collateral and Patellar Ligaments

① quadriceps femoris tendon

② lateral meniscus

③ tibial tuberosity

④ lateral collateral lig.

⑤ lateral femoral condyle

⑥ lateral epicondyle

⑦ medial epicondyle

⑧ medial meniscus

⑨ medial collateral lig.

⑩ tibia, medial surface

⑪ patellar lig.

⑫ femoropatellar joint

✱ Collateral ligs. are typical stabilizing components of flexion–extension joints. In the knee, the medial collateral lig. is attached to both the capsule and the medial meniscus, whereas the lateral collateral lig. has no direct contact with either the capsule or the lateral meniscus. Both ligaments are taut when the knee is extended and stabilize the joint in the coronal plane.

Menisci in the Knee Joint

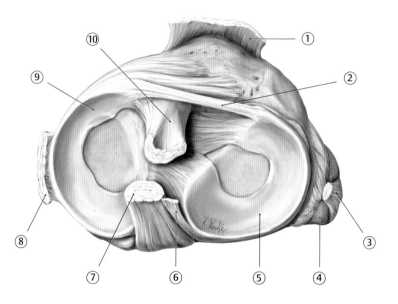

? A traumatic tear of the medial meniscus is often accompanied by damage to which other structures of the knee?

Menisci in the Knee Joint

① patellar lig.

② transverse lig. of knee

③ lateral collateral lig.

④ head of fibula

⑤ lateral meniscus

⑥ posterior meniscofemoral lig.

⑦ posterior cruciate lig.

⑧ medial collateral lig.

⑨ medial meniscus

⑩ anterior cruciate lig.

⚠ Trauma to the knee, especially a lateral blow, often results in a triad of injury that includes a tearing of the medial meniscus and rupture of the medial collateral and anterior cruciate ligs.

Fig. 32.8A. From *Atlas of Anatomy, Third Edition*, p. 433.

Cruciate and Collateral Ligaments, Anterior View

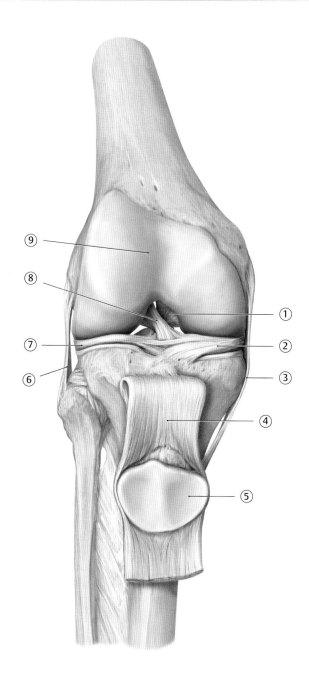

Cruciate and Collateral Ligaments, Anterior View

1. posterior cruciate lig.
2. medial meniscus
3. medial collateral lig.
4. patellar lig. (reflected)
5. patella
6. lateral collateral lig.
7. anterior cruciate lig.
8. patellar surface of femur

Fig. 32.10A. From *Atlas of Anatomy, Third Edition*, p. 434.

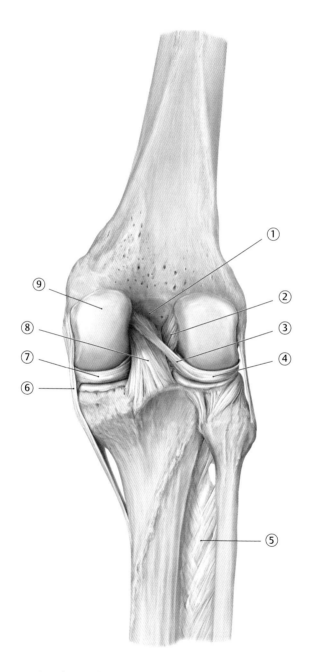

Cruciate and Collateral Ligaments, Posterior View

① intercondylar notch

② anterior cruciate lig.

③ posterior meniscofemoral lig.

④ lateral meniscus

⑤ interosseous membrane

⑥ medial collateral lig.

⑦ medial meniscus

⑧ posterior cruciate lig.

⑨ medial femoral condyle

Fig. 32.10B. From *Atlas of Anatomy, Third Edition*, p. 434.

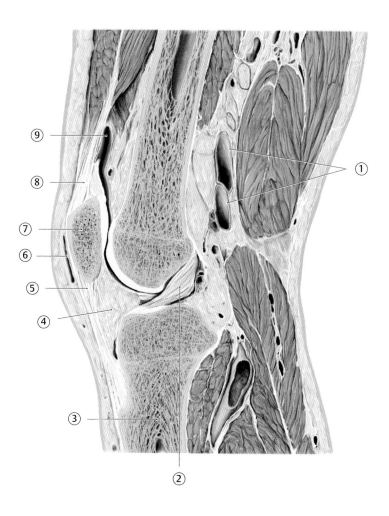

Midsagittal Section through the Knee

① popliteal v. and a.

② anterior cruciate lig.

③ tibia

④ infrapatellar fat pad

⑤ patellar lig.

⑥ prepatellar bursa

⑦ patella

⑧ quadriceps tendon

⑨ suprapatellar pouch

Fig. 32.17. From *Atlas of Anatomy, Third Edition*, p. 437.

Muscles of the Anterior Compartment of the Leg

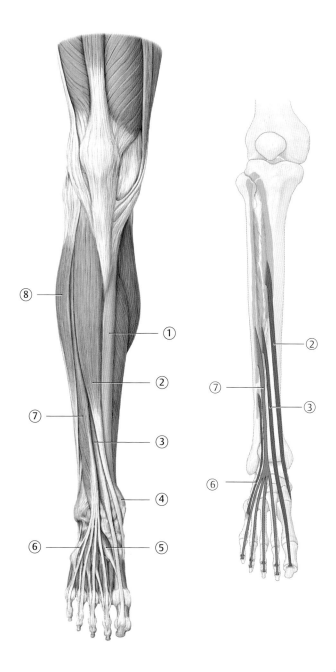

Muscles of the Anterior Compartment of the Leg

① tibia

② tibialis anterior

③ extensor hallucis

④ medial malleolus

⑤ extensor hallucis brevis

⑥ fibularis tertius

⑦ extensor digitorum longus

⑧ fibularis longus

Muscle	Origin	Insertion	Innervation	Action
Tibialis anterior	Tibia (upper two thirds of the lateral surface), interosseous membrane, and superficial crural fascia (highest part)	Medial cuneiform (medial and plantar surface), 1st metatarsal (medial base)	Deep fibular n. (L4, L5)	• Talocrural joint: Dorsiflexion • Subtalar joint: Inversion (supination)
Extensor hallucis longus	Fibula (middle third of the medial surface), interosseous membrane	1st toe (at the dorsal aponeurosis at the base of its distal phalanx)	Deep fibular n. (L4, L5)	• Talocrural joint: Dorsiflexion • Subtalar joint: Active in both eversion and inversion (pronation/supination), depending on the initial position of the foot • Extends the MTP and IP joints of the big toe
Extensor digitorum longus	Fibula (head and medial surface), tibia (lateral condyle), and interosseous membrane	2nd–5th toes (at the dorsal aponeuroses at the bases of the distal phalanges)	Deep fibular n. (L4, L5)	• Talocrural joint: Dorsiflexion • Subtalar joint: Eversion (pronation) • Extends the MTP and IP joints of the 2nd–5th toes
Fibularis tertius	Distal fibula (anterior border)	5th metatarsal (base)	Deep fibular n. (L4, L5)	• Talocrural joint: Dorsiflexion • Subtalar joint: Eversion (pronation)

IP, interphalangeal; MTP, metatarsophalangeal.

Fig. 32.22A, Fig. 32.18A. From *Atlas of Anatomy, Third Edition*, pp. 443, 438.

Muscles of the Lateral Compartment of the Leg

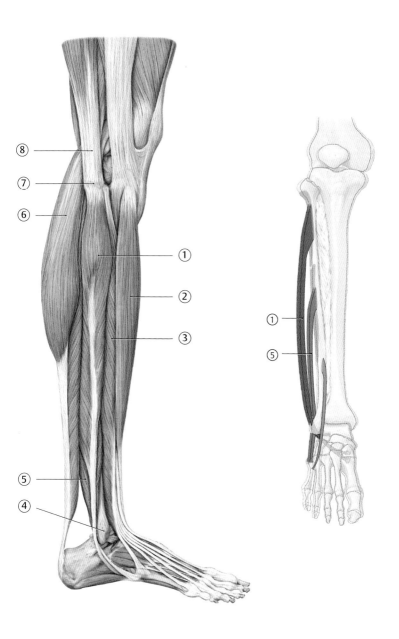

Muscles of the Lateral Compartment of the Leg

① fibularis longus

② tibialis anterior

③ extensor digitorum longus

④ lateral malleolus

⑤ fibularis brevis

⑥ gastrocnemius, lateral head

⑦ head of fibula

⑧ biceps femoris, common tendon of insertion

Muscle	Origin	Insertion	Innervation	Action
Fibularis longus	Fibula (head and proximal two thirds of the lateral surface, arising partly from the intermuscular septa)	Medial cuneiform (plantar side), 1st metatarsal (base)	Superficial fibular n. (L5, S1)	• Talocrural joint: Plantar flexion • Subtalar joint: Eversion (pronation) • Supports the transverse arch of the foot
Fibularis brevis	Fibula (distal half of the lateral surface), intermuscular septa	5th metatarsal (tuberosity at the base, with an occasional division to the dorsal aponeurosis of the 5th toe)		• Talocrural joint: Plantar flexion • Subtalar joint: Eversion (pronation)

Fig. 32.19, Fig. 32.21A. From *Atlas of Anatomy, Third Edition*, pp. 439, 442.

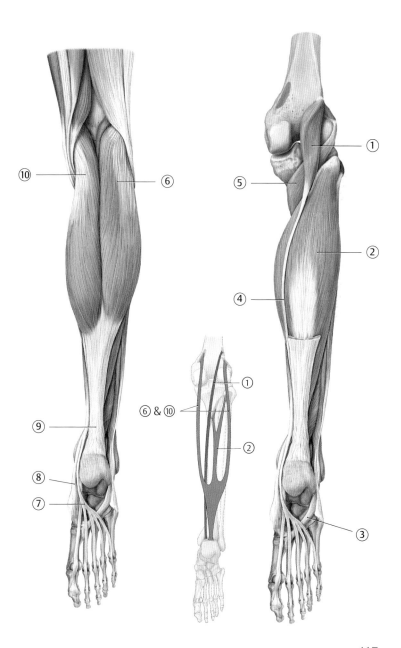

Muscles of the Superficial Posterior Compartment of the Leg

① plantaris

② soleus

③ fibularis longus

④ plantaris tendon

⑤ popliteus

⑥ gastrocnemius, lateral head

⑦ flexor digitorum longus

⑧ tibialis posterior

⑨ calcaneal (Achilles) tendon

⑩ gastrocnemius, medial head

Muscle		Origin	Insertion	Innervation	Action
Triceps surae	Gastrocnemius	Femur (medial head: superior posterior part of the medial femoral condyle; lateral head: lateral surface of lateral femoral condyle)	Calcaneal tuberosity via the calcaneal (Achilles) tendon	Tibial n. (S1, S2)	• Talocrural joint: Plantar flexion when knee is extended (gastrocnemius) • Knee joint: Flexion (gastrocnemius) • Talocrural joint: Plantar flexion (soleus)
	Soleus	Fibula (head and neck, posterior surface), tibia (soleal line via a tendinous arch)			
Plantaris		Femur (lateral epicondyle, proximal to lateral head of gastrocnemius)	Calcaneal tuberosity		Negligible; May act with gastrocnemius in plantar flexion

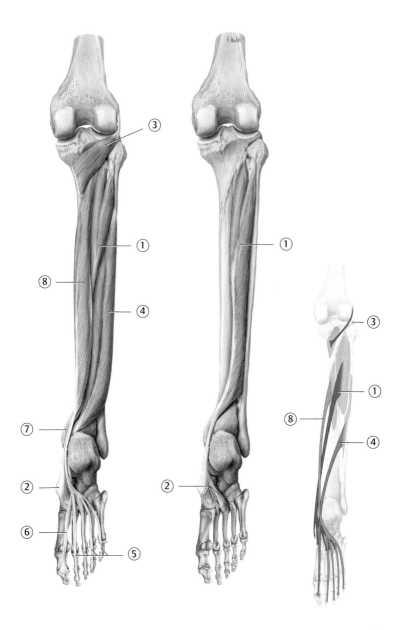

Muscles of the Deep Posterior Compartment of the Leg

① tibialis posterior

② tibialis posterior tendon

③ popliteus

④ flexor hallucis longus

⑤ flexor digitorum longus tendons

⑥ flexor hallucis longus tendon

⑦ medial malleolus

⑧ flexor digitorum longus

Muscle	Origin	Insertion	Innervation	Action
Tibialis posterior	Interosseous membrane, adjacent borders of tibia and fibula	Navicular tuberosity; cuneiforms (medial, intermediate, and lateral); 2nd–4th metatarsals (bases)	Tibial n. (L4, L5)	• Talocrural joint: Plantar flexion • Subtalar joint: Inversion (supination) • Supports the longitudinal and transverse arches
Flexor digitorum longus	Tibia (middle third of posterior surface)	2nd–5th distal phalanges (bases)	Tibial n. (L5–S2)	• Talocrural joint: Plantar flexion • Subtalar joint: Inversion (supination) • MTP and IP joints of the 2nd–5th toes: plantar flexion
Flexor hallucis longus	Fibula (distal two thirds of posterior surface), adjacent interosseous membrane	1st distal phalanx (base)		• Talocrural joint: Plantar flexion • Subtalar joint: Inversion (supination) • MTP and IP joints of the 1st toe: Plantar flexion • Supports the medial longitudinal arch
Popliteus	Lateral femoral condyle, posterior horn of the lateral meniscus	Posterior tibial surface (above the origin at the soleus)	Tibial n. (L4–S1)	Knee joint: Flexes and unlocks the knee by internally rotating the femur on the fixed tibia 5°

IP, interphalangeal; MTP, metatarsophalangeal.

Fig. 32.24A,B,C. From *Atlas of Anatomy, Third Edition*, p. 445.

Bones of the Foot: Right Foot, Dorsal View

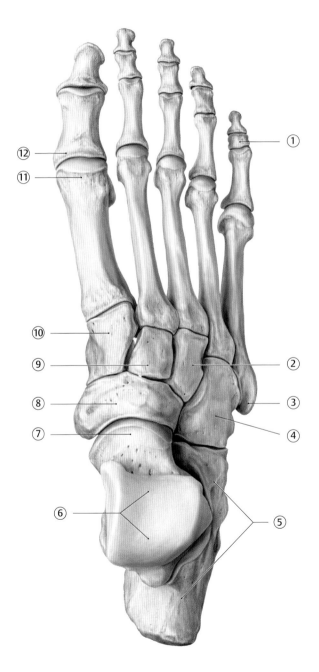

Bones of the Foot: Right Foot, Dorsal View

① 5th middle phalanx
② lateral cuneiform
③ tuberosity of 5th metatarsal
④ cuboid
⑤ calcaneus
⑥ trochlea of talus
⑦ head of talus
⑧ navicular
⑨ intermediate cuneiform
⑩ medial cuneiform
⑪ head of 1st metatarsal
⑫ base of 1st proximal phalanx

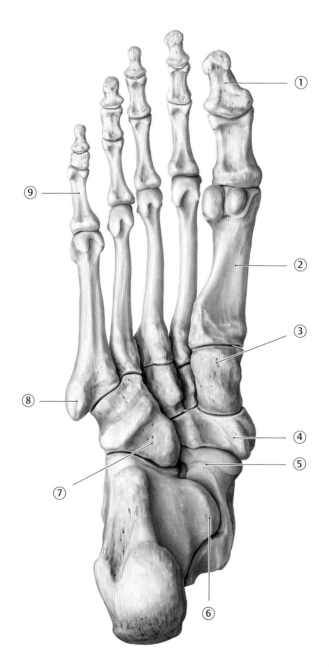

Bones of the Foot: Right Foot, Plantar View

① 1st distal phalanx

② 1st metatarsal

③ medial cuneiform

④ navicular

⑤ head of talus

⑥ sustentaculum tali

⑦ cuboid

⑧ tuberosity of 5th metatarsal

⑨ 5th proximal phalanx

Fig. 33.2C. From *Atlas of Anatomy, Third Edition*, p. 447.

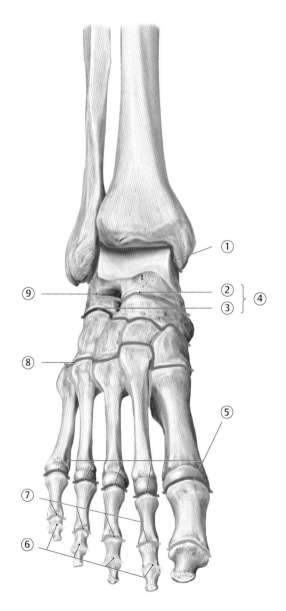

Why are ankle injuries more likely to occur when the foot is in plantar flexion?

Joints of the Ankle and Foot

①   talocrural (ankle) joint
②   talonavicular joint
③   calcaneocuboid joint
④   transverse tarsal joint
⑤   metatarsophalangeal joints
⑥   distal interphalangeal joints
⑦   proximal interphalangeal joints
⑧   tarsometatarsal joints
⑨   subtalar joint

⚠ Ankle injuries are more likely to occur when the joint is in plantar flexion because the trochlea of the talus is narrower posteriorly, so there is laxity within the tibiofibular mortise during plantar flexion. This results in greater instability and increased vulnerability to injury.

Fig. 33.3A. From *Atlas of Anatomy, Third Edition*, p. 448.

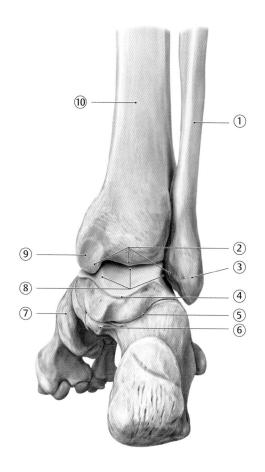

What movements occur at the talocrural and subtalar joints?

Talocrural and Subtalar Joints, Posterior View

①   fibula

②   ankle mortise

③   lateral malleolus

④   talus

⑤   subtalar (talocalcaneal) joint

⑥   sustentaculum tali

⑦   navicular

⑧   talocrural joint

⑨   medial malleolus

⑩   tibia

❗ The articulation between the trochlea of the talus and tibiofibular mortise allows only flexion and extension movements, whereas most inversion and eversion of the foot occurs at the subtalar joint.

Fig. 33.6A. From *Atlas of Anatomy, Third Edition*, p. 450.

Sagittal Section through the Foot

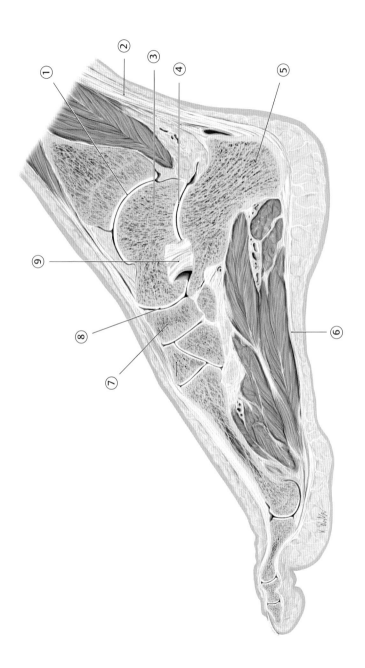

Sagittal Section through the Foot

① talocrural joint
② calcaneal (Achilles) tendon
③ talus
④ talocalcaneal joint (posterior compartment of subtalar joint)
⑤ calcaneus
⑥ plantar aponeurosis
⑦ navicular
⑧ talocalcaneonavicular joint (anterior compartment of subtalar joint)
⑨ interosseous talocalcaneal lig.

Fig. 33.7. From *Atlas of Anatomy, Third Edition*, p. 451.

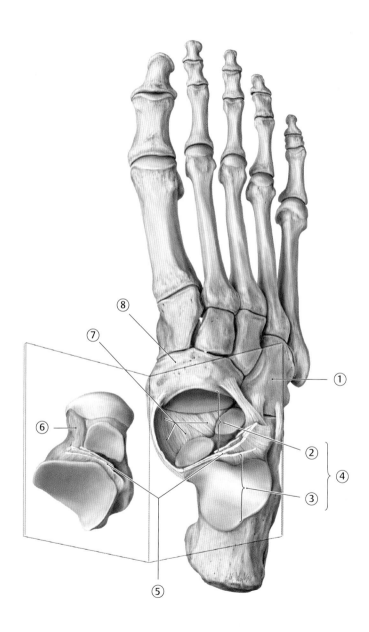

Subtalar Joint and Ligaments

① cuboid

② anterior compartment

③ posterior compartment

④ subtalar joint

⑤ interosseous talocalcaneal lig.

⑥ talus

⑦ plantar calcaneonavicular lig.

⑧ navicular

The plantar calcaneonavicular lig., also known as the "spring" lig., supports the head of the talus where it forms the highest point of the medial arch of the foot.

Fig. 33.9A. From *Atlas of Anatomy, Third Edition*, p. 452.

Ligaments of the Ankle and Foot, Medial View

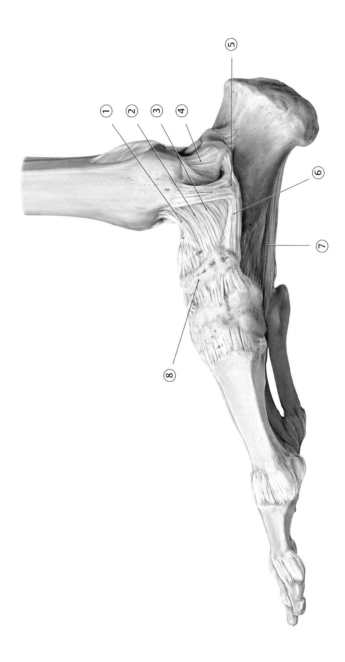

Ligaments of the Ankle and Foot, Medial View

① deltoid lig., anterior tibiotalar part
② deltoid lig., tibionavicular part
③ deltoid lig., tibiocalcaneal part
④ deltoid lig., posterior tibiotalar part
⑤ sustentaculum tali
⑥ plantar calcaneonavicular lig.
⑦ long plantar lig.
⑧ navicular

Fig. 33.11C. From *Atlas of Anatomy, Third Edition*, p. 455.

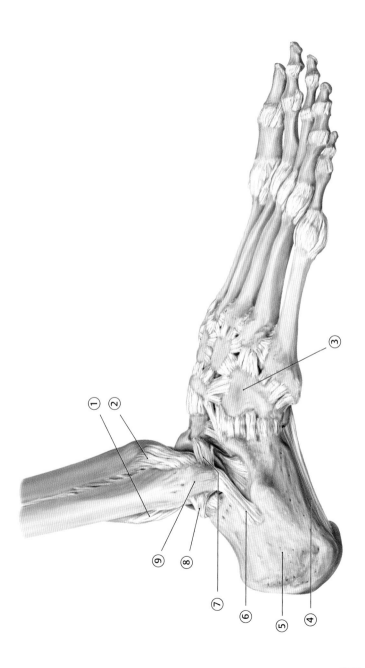

Ligaments of the Ankle and Foot, Lateral View

①   posterior tibiofibular lig.

②   anterior tibiofibular lig.

③   cuboid

④   long plantar lig.

⑤   calcaneus

⑥   calcaneofibular lig.

⑦   anterior talofibular lig.

⑧   posterior talofibular lig.

⑨   lateral malleolus

Fig. 33.11D. From *Atlas of Anatomy, Third Edition*, p. 455.

Plantar Aponeurosis

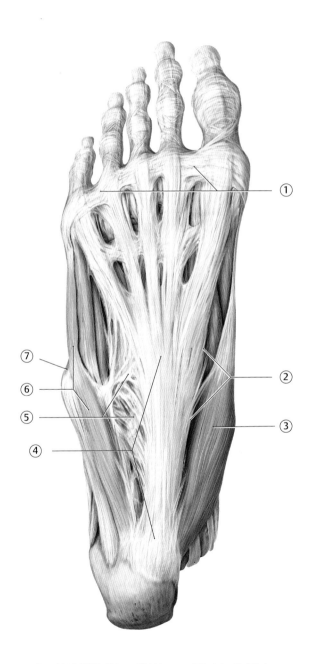

Plantar Aponeurosis

1. superficial transverse metatarsal lig.
2. medial plantar septum
3. abductor hallucis
4. plantar aponeurosis
5. lateral plantar septum
6. abductor digiti minimi
7. tuberosity of 5th metatarsal

✳ The plantar aponeurosis attaches tightly to the sole of the foot and acts as an important support for the arches of the foot. Plantar fasciitis, a painful condition that commonly afflicts runners, results from inflammation of the aponeurosis.

Fig. 33.15. From *Atlas of Anatomy, Third Edition*, p. 458.

Superficial Intrinsic Muscles of the Sole of the Foot

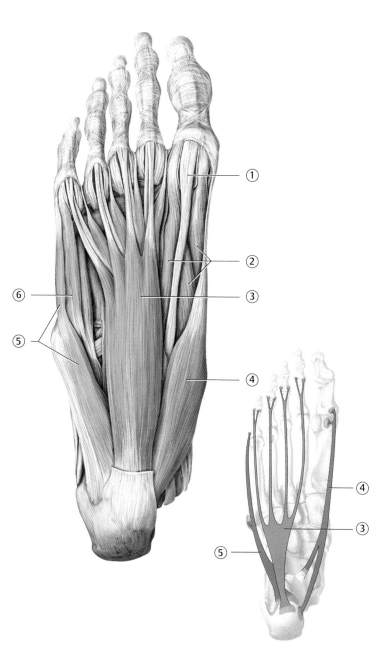

Superficial Intrinsic Muscles of the Sole of the Foot

① flexor hallucis longus tendon

② flexor hallucis brevis

③ flexor digitorum brevis

④ abductor hallucis

⑤ abductor digiti minimi

⑥ flexor digiti minimi brevis

Muscle	Origin	Insertion	Innervation	Action
Abductor hallucis	Calcaneal tuberosity (medial process); Flexor retinaculum, plantar aponeurosis	1st toe (base of proximal phalanx via the medial sesamoid)	Medial plantar n. (S1, S2)	• 1st MTP joint: Flexion and abduction of the 1st toe • Supports the longitudinal arch
Flexor digitorum brevis	Calcaneal tuberosity (medial tubercle), plantar aponeurosis	2nd–5th toes (sides of middle phalanges)		• Flexes the MTP and PIP joints of the 2nd–5th toes • Supports the longitudinal arch
Abductor digiti minimi		5th toe (base of proximal phalanx), 5th metatarsal (at tuberosity)	Lateral plantar n. (S1–S3)	• Flexes the MTP joint of the 5th toe • Abducts the 5th toe • Supports the longitudinal arch

MTP, metatarsophalangeal; PIP, proximal interphalangeal.

Fig. 33.16A, Fig. 33.20A. From *Atlas of Anatomy, Third Edition*, pp. 458, 463.

Deep Intrinsic Muscles of the Sole of the Foot I

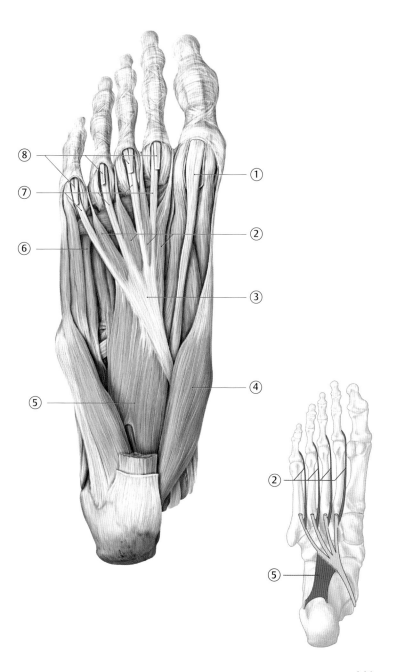

Deep Intrinsic Muscles of the Sole of the Foot I

① flexor halluces longus tendon

② lumbricals

③ flexor digitorum longus

④ abductor halluces

⑤ quadratus plantae

⑥ 3rd plantar interosseous

⑦ flexor digitorum longus tendons

⑧ flexor digitorum brevis tendons

Muscle	Origin	Insertion	Innervation	Action
Quadratus plantae	Calcaneal tuberosity (medial and plantar borders on plantar side)	Flexor digitorum longus tendon (lateral border)	Lateral plantar n. (S1–S3)	Redirects and augments the pull of flexor digitorum longus
Lumbricals (four muscles)	Flexor digitorum longus tendons (medial borders)	2nd–5th toes (at dorsal aponeuroses)	1st lumbrical: Medial plantar n. (S2, S3) 2nd–4th lumbrical: Lateral plantar n. (S2, S3)	• Flexes the MTP joints of 2nd–5th toes • Extension of IP joints of 2nd–5th toes • Adducts 2nd–5th toes toward the big toe
IP, interphalangeal; MTP, metatarsophalangeal.				

Deep Intrinsic Muscles of the Sole of the Foot II

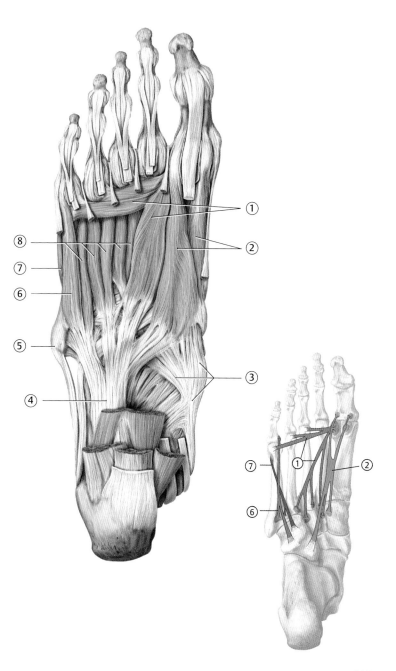

Deep Intrinsic Muscles of the Sole of the Foot II

① adductor hallucis, transverse and oblique heads

② flexor hallucis brevis, medial and lateral heads

③ tibialis posterior tendon

④ long plantar lig.

⑤ tuberosity of 5th metatarsal

⑥ flexor digiti minimi brevis

⑦ opponens digiti minimi

⑧ plantar and dorsal interossei

Muscle	Origin	Insertion	Innervation	Action
Flexor hallucis brevis	Cuboid, lateral cuneiforms, and plantar calcaneocuboid lig.	1st toe (at base of proximal phalanx via medial and lateral sesamoids)	Medial head: Medial plantar n. (S1, S2) Lateral head: Lateral plantar n. (S1, S2)	• Flexes the first MTP joint • Supports the longitudinal arch
Adductor hallucis	Oblique head: 2nd–4th metatarsals (at bases) cuboid and lateral cuneiforms — Transverse head: MTP joints of 3rd–5th toes, deep transverse metatarsal lig.	1st proximal phalanx (at base, by a common tendon via the lateral sesamoid)	Lateral plantar n., deep branch (S2, S3)	• Flexes the first MTP joint • Adducts big toe • Transverse head: Supports transverse arch • Oblique head: Supports longitudinal arch
Flexor digiti minimi brevis	5th metatarsal (base), long plantar lig.	5th toe (base of proximal phalanx)	Lateral plantar n., superficial branch (S2, S3)	Flexes the MTP joint of the little toe
Opponens digiti minimi*	Long plantar lig.; fibularis longus (at plantar tendon sheath)	5th metatarsal		Pulls 5th metatarsal in plantar and medial direction

*May be absent. IP, interphalangeal; MTP, metatarsophalangeal.

Fig. 33.16C, Fig. 33.21B. From *Atlas of Anatomy, Third Edition*, pp. 459, 464.

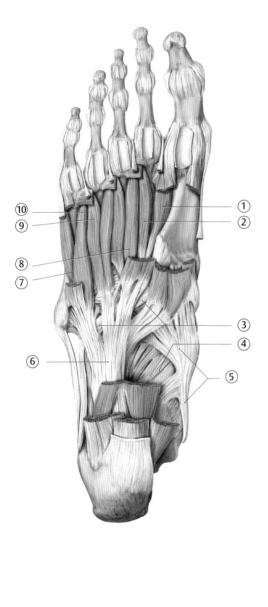

⑩

⑨

⑧

⑦

⑥

①

②

③

④

⑤

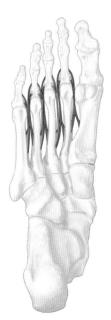

Deep Intrinsic Muscles of the Sole of the Foot III

① 1st dorsal interosseous

② 2nd dorsal interosseous

③ fibularis longus tendon

④ plantar calcaneonavicular lig.

⑤ tibialis posterior tendon

⑥ long plantar lig.

⑦ opponens digiti minimi

⑧ 1st plantar interosseous

⑨ 4th dorsal interosseous

⑩ 3rd plantar interosseous

Muscle	Origin	Insertion	Innervation	Action
Plantar interossei (three muscles)	3rd–5th metatarsals (medial border)	3rd–5th toes (medial base of proximal phalanx)	Lateral plantar n. (S2, S3)	• Flexes the MTP joints of 3rd–5th toes • Extension of IP joints of 3rd–5th toes • Adducts 3rd–5th toes toward 2nd toe
Dorsal interossei (four muscles)	1st–5th metatarsals (by two heads on opposing sides)	1st interosseus: 2nd proximal phalanx (medial base) 2nd–4th interossei: 2nd–4th proximal phalanges (lateral base), 2nd–4th toes (at dorsal aponeuroses)		• Flexes the MTP joints of 2nd–4th toes • Extension of IP joints of 2nd–4th toes • Abducts 3rd–4th toes from 2nd toe
IP, interphalangeal; MTP, metatarsophalangeal.				

Fig. 33.17A, Fig. 33.21C. From *Atlas of Anatomy, Third Edition*, pp. 460, 464.

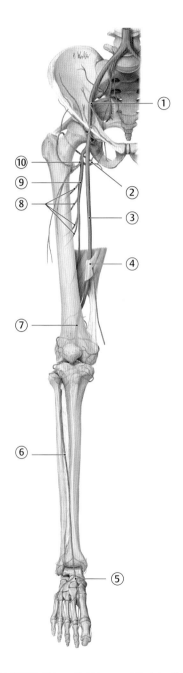

Arteries of the Lower Limb, Anterior View

① external iliac a.

② medial circumflex femoral a.

③ femoral a.

④ adductor canal (with adductor magnus)

⑤ dorsal pedal a.

⑥ anterior tibial a.

⑦ popliteal a.

⑧ 1st–4th perforating aa.

⑨ deep a. of thigh

⑩ lateral femoral circumflex femoral a.

Fig. 34.1A. From *Atlas of Anatomy, Third Edition*, p. 466.

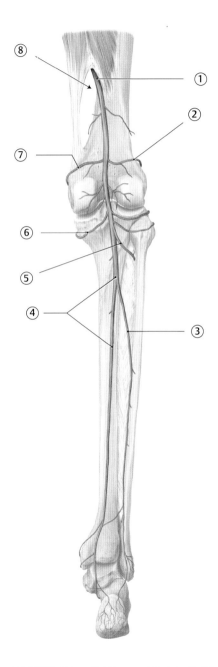

Arteries of the Lower Limb, Posterior View

① popliteal a.

② lateral superior genicular a.

③ fibular a.

④ posterior tibial a.

⑤ anterior tibial a.

⑥ medial inferior genicular a.

⑦ medial superior genicular a.

⑧ adductor hiatus

Fig. 34.1B. From *Atlas of Anatomy, Third Edition*, p. 466.

Veins of the Lower Limb

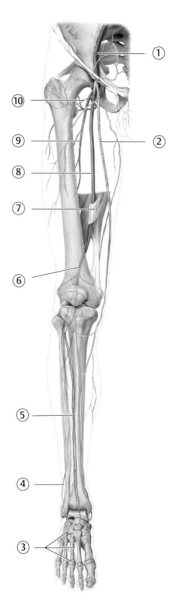

❓ How does the flow of blood from the lower limb counter the downward force of gravity?

Veins of the Lower Limb

① external iliac v.

② great saphenous v.

③ dorsal venous network of foot

④ small saphenous v.

⑤ anterior tibial vv.

⑥ popliteal v.

⑦ adductor canal

⑧ femoral v.

⑨ deep v. of thigh

⑩ lateral circumflex femoral v.

As in the upper limb, venous drainage in the lower limb flows from the superficial veins into the deep venous system. In both deep and superficial systems, the upward flow of blood is assisted by the presence of venous valves (over 20 in the great saphenous v.), the pulsing of accompanying arteries and contraction of surrounding muscles.

Fig. 34.6A. From *Atlas of Anatomy, Third Edition*, p. 468.

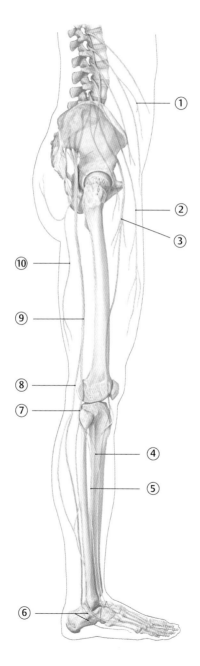

Nerves of the Lumbosacral Plexus

① iliohypogastric n.

② lateral cutaneous n. of thigh

③ femoral n.

④ deep fibular n.

⑤ superficial fibular n.

⑥ medial and lateral plantar nn.

⑦ common fibular n.

⑧ tibial n.

⑨ sciatic n.

⑩ posterior cutaneous n. of thigh

Lumbar plexus		
Iliohypogastric n.		L1
Ilioinguinal n.		L1
Genitofemoral n.		L1–L2
Lateral cutaneous n. of the thigh		L2–L3
Obturator n.		L2–L4
Femoral n.		
Sacral plexus		
Superior gluteal n.		L4–S1
Inferior gluteal n.		L5–S2
Posterior cutaneous n. of the thigh		S1–S3
Sciatic n.	Common fibular n.	L4–S2
	Tibial n.	L4–S3
Pudendal n.		S2–S4

Table 34.1. From *Atlas of Anatomy*, *Third Edition*, p. 470.

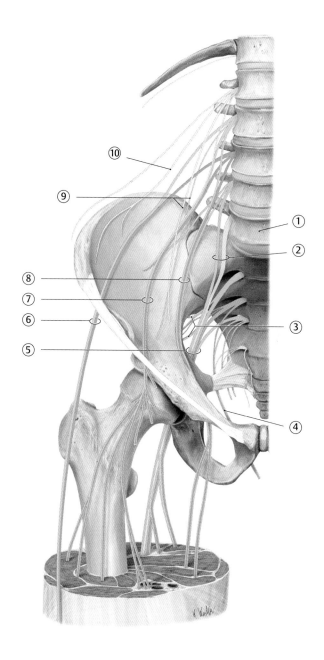

Lumbosacral Plexus In Situ

① L5 vertebra
② lumbosacral trunk
③ superior and inferior gluteal nn.
④ pudendal n.
⑤ sciatic n.
⑥ lateral cutaneous n. of thigh
⑦ femoral n.
⑧ obturator n.
⑨ genitofemoral n.
⑩ ilioinguinal n.

Muscles of the lower limb are innervated primarily by branches of the sacral plexus (L4–S3). Only the anterior and medial thigh muscles are innervated by branches (femoral and obturator nn.) of the lumbar plexus (L1–L4).

Fig. 34.11. From *Atlas of Anatomy, Third Edition*, p. 471.

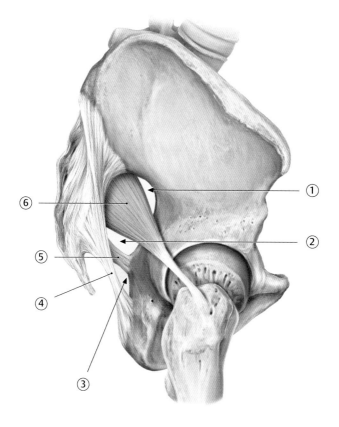

Sciatic Foramina

① greater sciatic foramen, suprapiriform part

② greater sciatic foramen, infrapiriform part

③ lesser sciatic foramen

④ sacrotuberous lig.

⑤ sacrospinous lig.

⑥ piriformis

Foramen		Transmitted structures	Boundaries
Greater sciatic foramen	Suprapiriform portion	Superior gluteal a., v., and n.	Greater sciatic notch Sacrospinous lig. Sacrum
	Infrapiriform portion	Inferior gluteal a., v., and n. Internal pudendal a. and v. Pudendal n. Sciatic n. Posterior cutaneous n. of the thigh	
Lesser sciatic foramen		Internal pudendal a. and v. Pudendal n. Obturator internus	Lesser sciatic notch Sacrospinous lig. Sacrotuberous lig.

Table 34.9. From *Atlas of Anatomy, Third Edition*, p. 485.

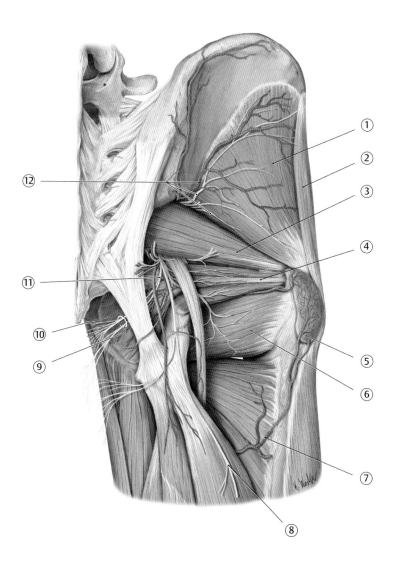

Neurovasculature of the Gluteal Region and Ischioanal Fossa

① gluteus minimus

② tensor fasciae latae

③ piriformis

④ obturator internus tendon

⑤ trochanteric bursa

⑥ quadratus femoris

⑦ 1st perforating a.

⑧ posterior cutaneous n. of thigh

⑨ pudendal canal

⑩ obturator internus

⑪ pudendal n.

⑫ superior gluteal a. and n.

Fig. 34.33. From *Atlas of Anatomy, Third Edition*, p. 485.

Femoral Triangle

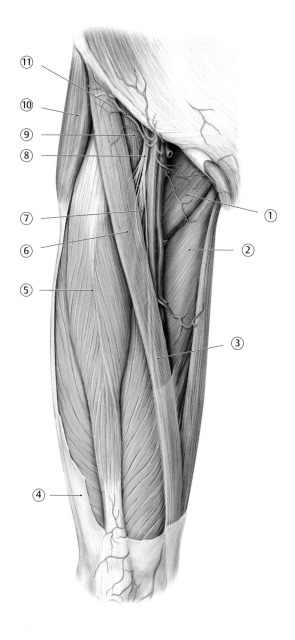

Femoral Triangle

1. pectineus
2. adductor longus
3. femoral a. and v. in adductor canal
4. fascia lata
5. rectus femoris
6. sartorius
7. deep a. of thigh
8. femoral n.
9. iliopsoas
10. tensor fasciae latae
11. superficial circumflex iliac a.

Fig. 34.34A. From *Atlas of Anatomy, Third Edition*, p. 486.

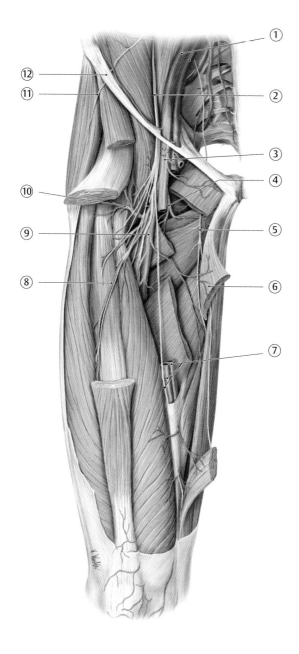

Neurovasculature of the Anterior Thigh

①   external iliac a. and v.

②   femoral n.

③   femoral a. and v.

④   medial circumflex femoral a.

⑤   obturator n.

⑥   adductor brevis

⑦   femoral a. and v., saphenous n.

⑧   lateral circumflex femoral a., descending branch.

⑨   deep a. of thigh

⑩   lateral circumflex femoral a., ascending branch

⑪   lateral cutaneous n. of thigh

⑫   inguinal lig.

Fig. 34.34B. From *Atlas of Anatomy, Third Edition*, p. 486.

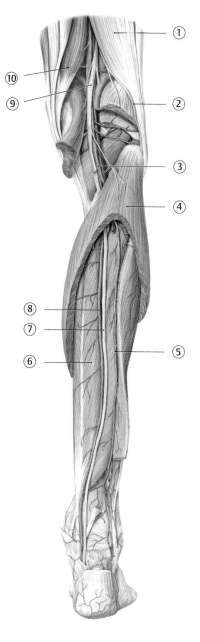

Neurovasculature of the Posterior Compartment of the Leg

① biceps femoris
② common fibular n.
③ popliteal a. and v.
④ soleus
⑤ fibular a.
⑥ flexor digitorum longus
⑦ tibial n.
⑧ posterior tibial a.
⑨ tibial n.
⑩ semimembranosus

Fig. 34.36. From *Atlas of Anatomy, Third Edition*, p. 488.

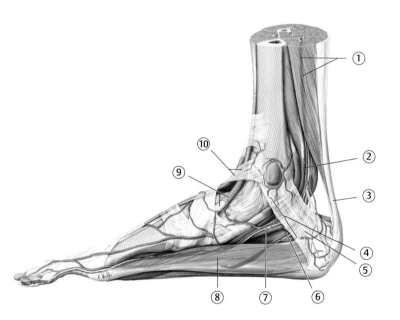

Ankle Region and the Tarsal Tunnel

① tibial n. and posterior tibial a.

② flexor digitorum longus

③ calcaneal (Achilles) tendon

④ tarsal tunnel

⑤ flexor retinaculum

⑥ lateral plantar a. and n.

⑦ medial plantar a. and n.

⑧ abductor hallucis

⑨ tibialis anterior

⑩ inferior extensor retinaculum

The tarsal tunnel is traversed by the long flexor tendons and the tibial n., a., and v. Tarsal tunnel syndrome, similar to carpal tunnel syndrome in the wrist, results from swelling of the synovial sheaths. Compression of the tibial nerve can cause pain, numbness, and tingling that radiates to the heel.

Fig. 34.38. From *Atlas of Anatomy, Third Edition*, p. 489.

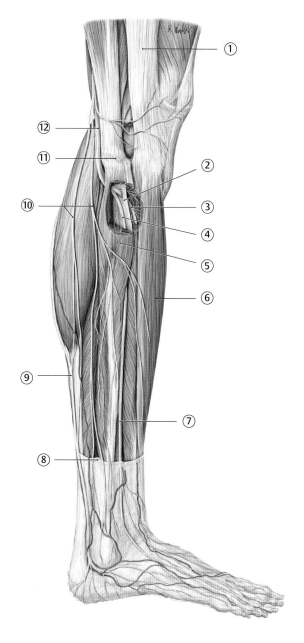

Neurovasculature of the Lateral Compartment of the Leg

1. iliotibial tract
2. anterior crural intermuscular septum
3. deep fibular n.
4. superficial fibular n.
5. fibularis longus
6. tibialis anterior
7. superficial fibular n.
8. deep fascia of leg
9. sural n.
10. lateral sural cutaneous n.
11. head of fibula
12. common fibular n.

Fig. 34.39. From *Atlas of Anatomy, Third Edition*, p. 490.

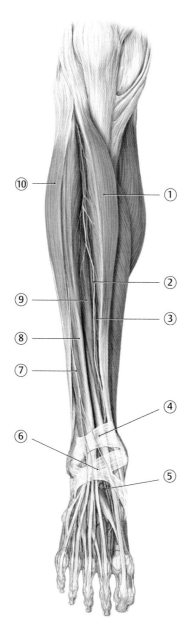

Neurovasculature of the Anterior Compartment of the Leg

① tibialis anterior
② deep fibular n.
③ anterior tibial a. and v.
④ superior extensor retinaculum
⑤ dorsalis pedis a.
⑥ inferior extensor retinaculum
⑦ superficial fibular n.
⑧ extensor digitorum longus
⑨ extensor hallucis longus
⑩ fibularis longus

Compartments of the Leg

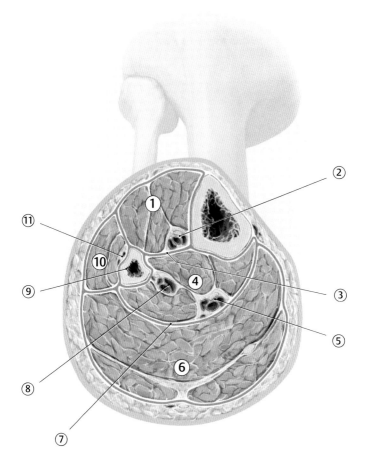

Compartments of the Leg

① anterior compartment
② deep fibular n., anterior tibial a. and v.
③ interosseous membrane
④ deep posterior compartment
⑤ tibial n., posterior tibial a. and v.
⑥ superficial posterior compartment
⑦ transverse intermuscular septum
⑧ fibular a. and v.
⑨ fibula
⑩ lateral compartment
⑪ superficial fibular n.

Compartment		Muscular contents	Neurovascular contents
Anterior compartment		Tibialis anterior	Deep fibular n.
		Extensor digitorum longus	Anterior tibial a. and v.
		Extensor halluces longus	
		Fibularis tertius	
Lateral compartment		Fibularis longus	Superficial fibular n.
		Fibularis brevis	
Posterior compartment	Superficial part	Triceps surae (gastrocnemius and soleus)	—
		Plantaris	
	Deep part	Tibialis posterior	Tibial n.
		Flexor digitorum longus	Posterior tibial a. and v.
		Flexor hallucis longus	Fibular a. and v.

Table 34.10. From *Atlas of Anatomy, Third Edition*, p. 490.

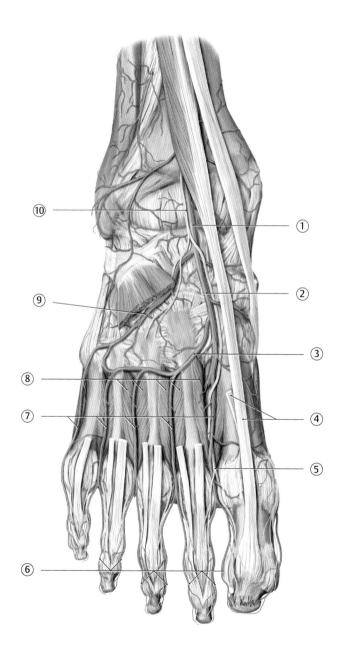

Neurovasculature of the Dorsum of the Foot

①   anterior tibial a.
②   dorsalis pedis a.
③   arcuate a.
④   extensor hallucis longus and brevis tendons
⑤   deep fibular n., cutaneous branch
⑥   dorsal digital aa.
⑦   dorsal metatarsal aa.
⑧   dorsal interossei
⑨   lateral tarsal a.
⑩   deep fibular n.

Fig. 34.40A. From *Atlas of Anatomy, Third Edition*, p. 491.

Neurovasculature of the Sole of the Foot

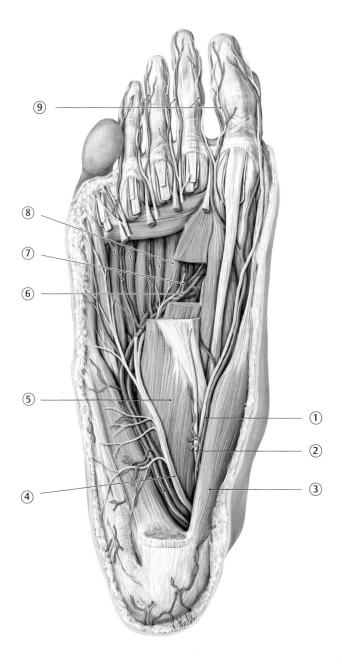

Neurovasculature of the Sole of the Foot

① medial plantar a.
② medial plantar n.
③ abductor hallucis
④ lateral plantar a., v., and n.
⑤ quadratus plantae
⑥ deep plantar arch
⑦ plantar metatarsal aa.
⑧ plantar interossei
⑨ proper plantar digital aa and nn.

Fig. 34.41. From *Atlas of Anatomy, Third Edition*, p. 492.

Head and Neck

(Continued)

Head and Neck

Regions of the Head and Neck

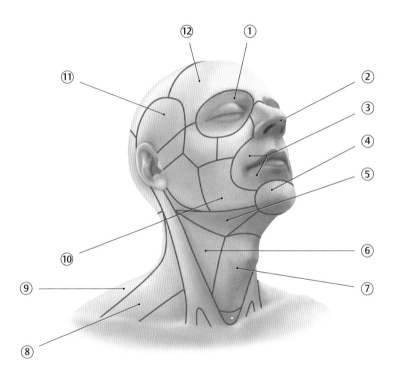

Regions of the Head and Neck

- ① orbital region
- ② nasal region
- ③ oral region
- ④ mental region
- ⑤ submandibular region
- ⑥ carotid triangle
- ⑦ muscular triangle
- ⑧ lateral cervical region
- ⑨ posterior cervical region
- ⑩ buccal region
- ⑪ temporal region
- ⑫ frontal region

Fig.36.1. From *Atlas of Anatomy, Third Edition*, p. 504.

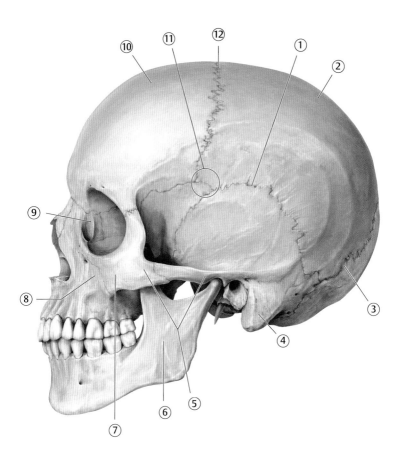

What is the significance of the pterion on the lateral skull?

Lateral Skull

1. squamous suture
2. parietal bone
3. lambdoid suture
4. mastoid process
5. zygomatic arch
6. mandible, ramus
7. zygomatic bone
8. maxilla, zygomatic process
9. lacrimal bone
10. frontal bone
11. pterion
12. coronal suture

❗ The pterion on the lateral skull marks the junction of the frontal, parietal, sphenoid, and temporal bones. Bone in this area is thin and overlies the middle meningeal artery, which runs deep to the skull in the epidural space. As a result of this relationship, skull fractures at the pterion can lead to life-threatening epidural hemorrhage.

Fig. 37.1. From *Atlas of Anatomy, Third Edition*, p. 506.

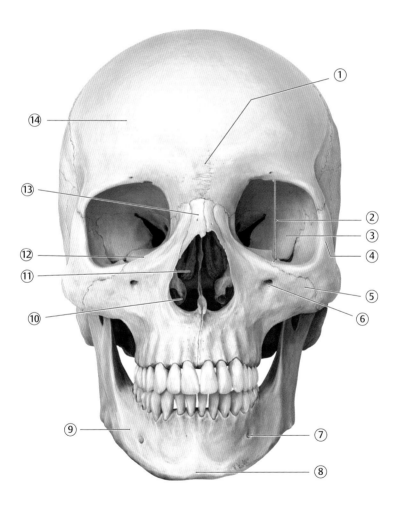

Anterior Skull

① glabella

② orbit

③ sphenoid bone, greater wing

④ zygomatic bone, frontal process

⑤ maxilla, zygomatic process

⑥ infraorbital foramen

⑦ mental foramen

⑧ mental protuberance

⑨ mandible, body

⑩ inferior nasal concha

⑪ ethmoid bone, middle nasal concha

⑫ infraorbital margin

⑬ nasal bone

⑭ frontal bone

The skull is subdivided into the neurocranium, which protects the brain, and the viscerocranium, which houses and protects the facial regions.

Fig. 37.2. From *Atlas of Anatomy, Third Edition*, p. 507.

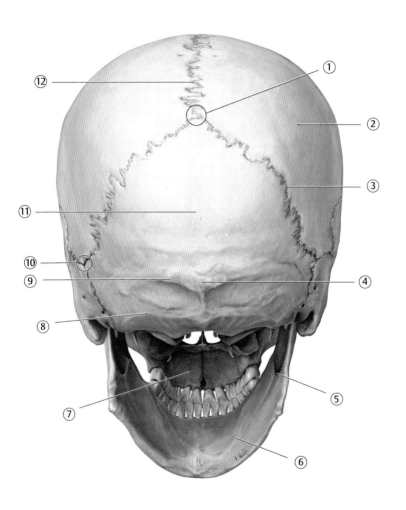

Posterior Skull

①   lambda
②   parietal bone
③   lambdoid suture
④   external occipital protuberance
⑤   mandibular foramen
⑥   mylohyoid line
⑦   maxilla, palatine process
⑧   inferior nuchal line
⑨   superior nuchal line
⑩   asterion
⑪   occipital bone
⑫   sagittal suture

Fig. 37.3. From *Atlas of Anatomy, Third Edition*, p. 508.

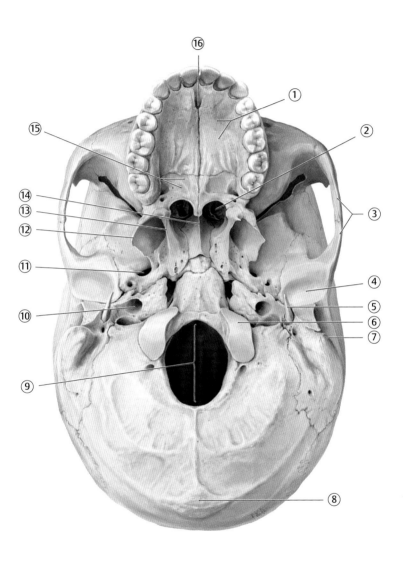

The medial and lateral pterygoid plates are components of which cranial bone?

Base of the Skull: Exterior

① palatine process

② choana

③ zygomatic arch

④ mandibular fossa

⑤ styloid process

⑥ occipital condyle

⑦ mastoid process

⑧ external occipital protuberance

⑨ foramen magnum

⑩ carotid canal

⑪ foramen ovale

⑫ lateral pterygoid plate

⑬ medial pterygoid plate

⑭ vomer

⑮ palatine bone

⑯ incisive foramen

❗ The medial and lateral pterygoid plates, processes of the sphenoid bone, are important attachment sites for muscles.

Fig. 37.6. From *Atlas of Anatomy, Third Edition*, p. 510.

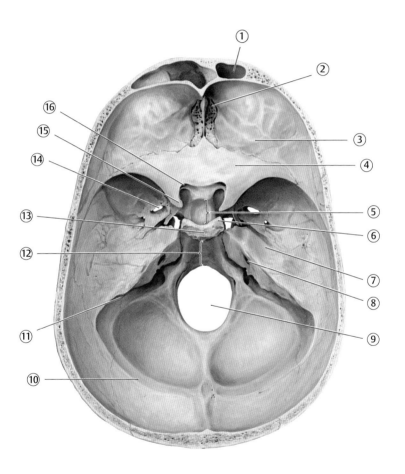

What are the boundaries of the middle cranial fossa?

Base of the Skull: Interior

① frontal sinus

② ethmoid bone, cribriform plate

③ frontal bone

④ sphenoid, lesser wing

⑤ sphenoid, hypophyseal fossa

⑥ posterior clinoid process

⑦ temporal bone, petrous part

⑧ internal acoustic meatus

⑨ foramen magnum

⑩ groove for transverse sinus

⑪ groove for sigmoid sinus

⑫ clivus

⑬ dorsum sellae

⑭ foramen ovale

⑮ anterior clinoid process

⑯ optic canal

❗ The floor of the cranial cavity is divided into three spaces, the anterior, middle, and posterior cranial fossae. The middle cranial fossa is formed anteriorly by the greater and lesser wings of the sphenoid bone, posteriorly and medially by the petrous part of the temporal bone, and laterally by the squamous part of the temporal bone.

Fig. 37.8. From *Atlas of Anatomy, Third Edition*, p. 511.

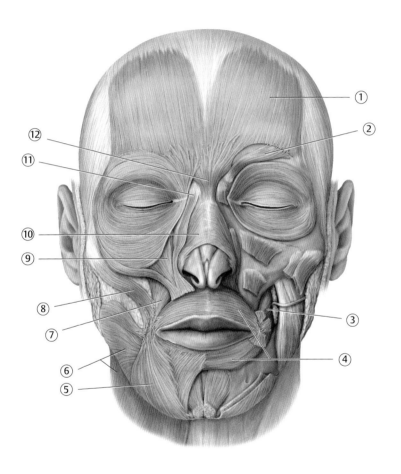

What is the innervation of muscles of facial expression?

Muscles of Facial Expression

① occipitofrontalis, frontal belly

② corrugator supercilii

③ buccinator

④ orbicularis oris

⑤ depressor anguli oris

⑥ platysma

⑦ levator anguli oris

⑧ zygomaticus major

⑨ levator labii superioris

⑩ nasalis

⑪ levator labii superioris alaeque nasi

⑫ procerus

⚠ All muscles of facial expression are innervated by the facial n. (CN VII). A lesion of the facial n. can lead to paralysis, i.e. drooping, of the ipsilateral face.

Fig. 38.1. From *Atlas of Anatomy, Third Edition*, p. 516.

Muscles of Mastication I

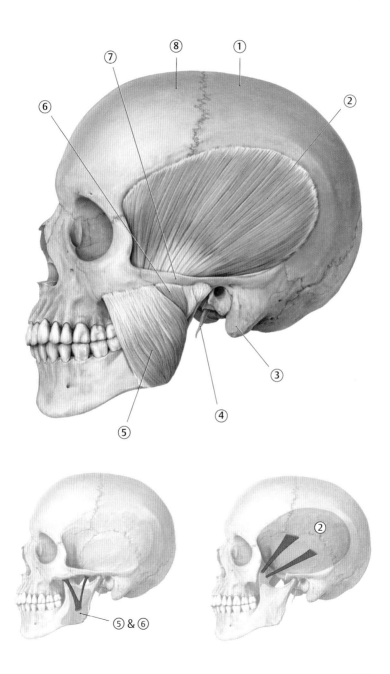

Muscles of Mastication I

① parietal bone
② temporalis
③ mastoid process
④ styloid process
⑤ masseter, superficial layer
⑥ masseter, deep layer
⑦ zygomatic arch
⑧ frontal bone

Muscle	Origin	Insertion	Innervation	Action
Masseter	Superficial layer: Zygomatic arch (anterior two thirds) / Deep layer: Zygomatic arch (posterior one third)	Mandibular angle (masseteric tuberosity)	Mandibular n. (CN V₃) via masseteric n.	Elevates (adducts) and protrudes mandible
Temporalis	Temporal fossa (inferior temporal line)	Coronoid process of mandible (apex and medial surface)	Mandibular n. (CN V₃) via deep temporal nn.	*Vertical fibers:* Elevate (adduct) mandible *Horizontal fibers:* Retract (retrude) mandible *Unilateral:* Lateral movement of mandible (chewing)

Fig. 38.11A,B, 38.12A. From *Atlas of Anatomy, Third Edition*, p. 522.

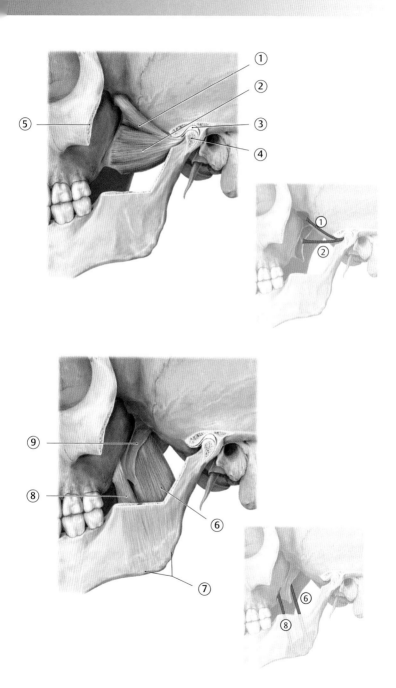

Muscles of Mastication II

① lateral pterygoid, superior head

② lateral pterygoid, inferior head

③ articular disk

④ condylar head

⑤ zygomatic arch

⑥ medial pterygoid, deep head

⑦ mandibular angle

⑧ medial pterygoid, superficial head

⑨ pterygoid process, lateral plate

Muscle		Origin	Insertion	Innervation	Action
Lateral pterygoid	Superior head	Greater wing of sphenoid bone (infratemporal crest)	Temporomandibular joint (articular disk)	Mandibular n. (CN V₃) via lateral pterygoid n.	*Bilateral:* Protrudes mandible (pulls articular disk forward) *Unilateral:* Lateral movements of mandible (chewing)
	Inferior head	Lateral pterygoid plate (lateral surface)	Mandible (condylar process)		
Medial pterygoid	Superficial head	Maxilla (tuberosity)	Pterygoid tuberosity on medial surface of the mandibular angle	Mandibular n. (CN V₃) via medial pterygoid n.	*Bilateral:* Elevates (adducts) mandible with masseter; contributes to protrusion. *Unilateral:* small grinding movements
	Deep head	Medial surface of lateral pterygoid plate and pterygoid fossa			

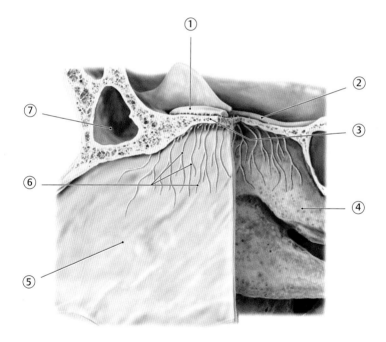

Cranial Nerves: CN I

① olfactory bulb
② olfactory tract
③ cribriform plate, ethmoid bone
④ superior concha
⑤ nasal septum
⑥ olfactory fibers (CN I)
⑦ frontal sinus

Fig. 39.3C. From *Atlas of Anatomy, Third Edition*, p. 526.

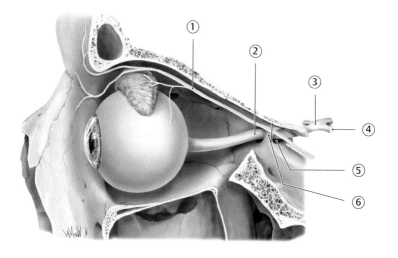

How does the course of the optic n. differ from other cranial nerves entering the orbit?

Cranial Nerves: CN II

① ophthalmic n. (CN V₁)

② optic n. (CN II) passing through optic canal

③ optic chiasm

④ optic tract

⑤ optic canal

⑥ superior orbital fissure

⚠ The optic n. passes through the optic canal. All other nerves of the orbit pass through the cavernous sinus and superior orbital fissure.

Fig. 39.4D. From *Atlas of Anatomy, Third Edition*, p. 527.

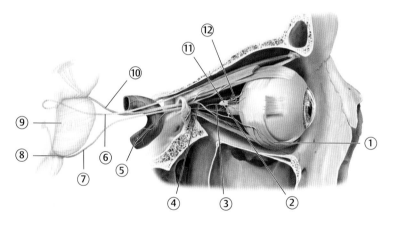

Which cranial nerves are involved in the pupillary light reflex?

Cranial Nerves: CN III, CN IV, CN VI

①   inferior oblique

②   parasympathetic root (CN III)

③   sympathetic root (via internal carotid plexus)

④   oculomotor n. (CN III), inferior division

⑤   internal carotid a. and plexus

⑥   trochlear n. (CN IV)

⑦   abducent n. (CN VI)

⑧   pontomedullary junction

⑨   pons

⑩   oculomotor n. (CN III)

⑪   ciliary ganglion

⑫   short ciliary nerves

! The pupillary light reflex, a rapid constriction of the pupil when exposed to light, involves the optic n. (CN II) as the afferent (sensory) limb and the oculomotor n. (CN III) as the efferent (motor) limb.

Fig. 39.6A. From *Atlas of Anatomy, Third Edition*, p. 529.

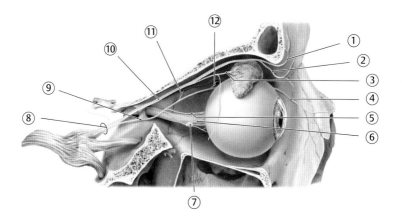

What type of nerve fibers are carried by the ophthalmic branch of the trigeminal nerve?

① supraorbital n.
② supratrochlear n.
③ lacrimal n.
④ infratrochlear n.
⑤ long ciliary nn.
⑥ short ciliary nn.
⑦ ciliary ganglion
⑧ ophthalmic division (CN V$_1$)
⑨ nasociliary n.
⑩ frontal n.
⑪ posterior ethmoidal n.
⑫ anterior ethmoidal n.

! The ophthalmic branch of the trigeminal nerve (CN V$_1$) carries only somatic sensory fibers.

Fig. 39.9A. From *Atlas of Anatomy, Third Edition*, p. 531.

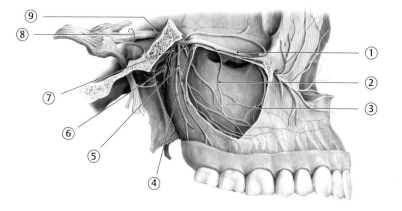

⑨
⑧
⑦
⑥
⑤
④
① ② ③

The maxillary division of the trigeminal nerve (CN V$_2$) carries postganglionic parasympathetic fibers that originate with which cranial nerves?

Cranial Nerves: CN V₂

① infraorbital n.
② middle superior alveolar n.
③ anterior superior alveolar branches
④ inferior orbital fissure
⑤ posterior superior alveolar nn.
⑥ pterygopalatine ganglion
⑦ ganglionic branches to pterygopalatine ganglion
⑧ maxillary division (CN V₂)
⑨ foramen rotundum

No parasympathetic nerves originate with the trigeminal nerve but some branches of its maxillary division help distribute postganglionic parasympathetic fibers that originate with the facial nerve (CN VII).

Fig. 39.9B. From *Atlas of Anatomy, Third Edition*, p. 531.

Cranial Nerves: CN V₃

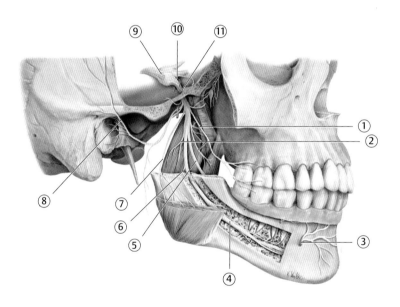

CN V₃ is the only division of the trigeminal nerve that carries motor fibers. Which muscles does it innervate?

Cranial Nerves: CN V₃

①   buccal n.

②   medial pterygoid nn.

③   mental n.

④   inferior alveolar n.

⑤   lingual n.

⑥   mylohyoid n.

⑦   masseteric n.

⑧   auriculotemporal n.

⑨   trigeminal ganglion

⑩   mandibular division (CN V₃)

⑪   foramen ovale

⚠ The mandibular division of the trigeminal n. (CN V₃) innervates the muscles of mastication (temporalis, masseter, medial pterygoid, and lateral pterygoid), in addition to the mylohyoid and anterior digastric on the floor of the mouth, the tensor veli palatini of the palate, and the tensor tympani of the middle ear.

Fig. 39.9C. From *Atlas of Anatomy, Third Edition*, p. 531.

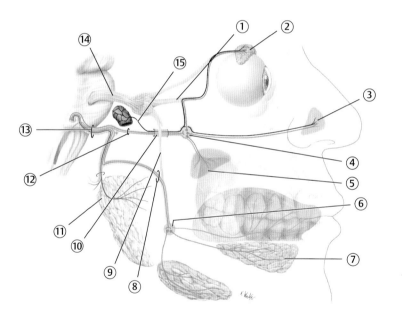

Cranial Nerves: CN VII

① maxillary division (CN V$_2$)
② lacrimal gland
③ nasal glands
④ pterygopalatine ganglion
⑤ taste buds of soft palate
⑥ submandibular gland
⑦ sublingual gland
⑧ chorda tympani
⑨ lingual n.
⑩ pterygoid canal with n. of pterygoid canal
⑪ parotid gland
⑫ greater petrosal n.
⑬ facial n. (CN VII)
⑭ trigeminal n. (CN V)
⑮ deep petrosal n.

Fig. 39.12. From *Atlas of Anatomy, Third Edition*, p. 533.

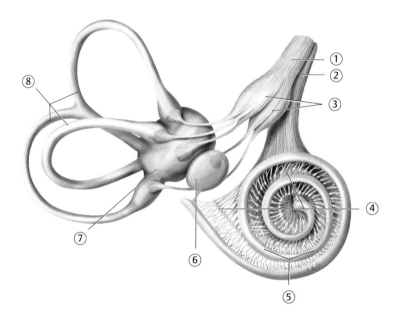

② What is the effect of a lesion to the vestibular or cochlear root of the vestibulocochlear n. (CN VIII)?

Cranial Nerves: CN VIII

①   vestibulocochlear n. (CN VIII), vestibular root

②   vestibulocochlear n. (CN VIII), cochlear root

③   vestibular ganglion

④   spiral ganglion

⑤   cochlear duct

⑥   saccule

⑦   utricle

⑧   semicircular ducts

The vestibulocochlear n. is a special somatic sensory nerve that consists of two roots. The vestibular root receives input from the semicircular canals, saccule, and utricle and transmits information concerning orientation in space. Injury to this nerve results in dizziness. The cochlear root transmits impulses from the organ of Corti of the cochlea. Injury to this nerve results in hearing loss.

Fig. 39.15. From *Atlas of Anatomy, Third Edition*, p. 535.

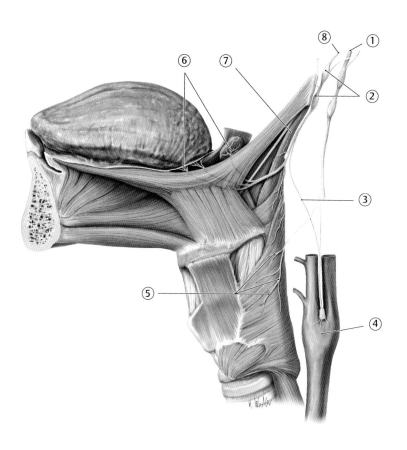

What is the pharyngeal plexus?

Cranial Nerves: CN IX

①   vagus n.

②   superior and inferior ganglia

③   branch to carotid sinus

④   carotid sinus

⑤   pharyngeal plexus

⑥   tonsillar and lingual branches

⑦   stylopharyngeus

⑧   glossopharyngeal n. (CN IX)

❗ The pharyngeal plexus is formed from fibers of the vagus n. (CN X) and the glossopharyngeal n. (CN IX). It innervates the muscles of the pharynx and the carotid sinus.

Fig. 39.18. From *Atlas of Anatomy, Third Edition*, p. 536.

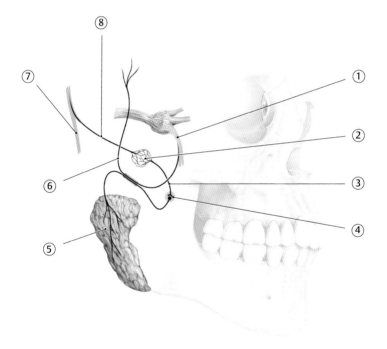

Cranial Nerves: CN IX Visceral Efferent

① mandibular division (CN V$_3$)

② tympanic plexus

③ lesser petrosal n.

④ otic ganglion

⑤ parotid gland

⑥ auriculotemporal n.

⑦ glossopharyngeal n. (CN IX)

⑧ tympanic n.

Fig. 39.20. From *Atlas of Anatomy, Third Edition*, p. 537.

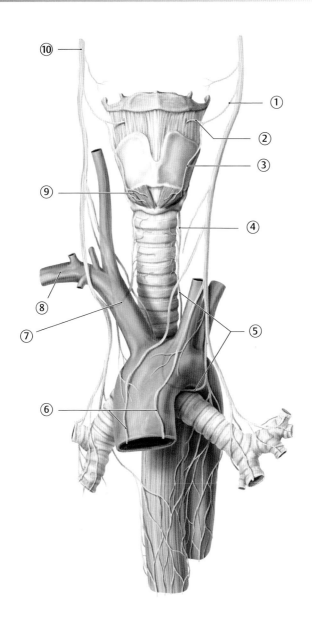

What kind of injury would be indicated by a patient who exhibits hoarseness following thyroid surgery?

Cranial Nerves: CN X

① superior laryngeal n.
② internal laryngeal n.
③ external laryngeal n.
④ left inferior laryngeal n.
⑤ left recurrent laryngeal n.
⑥ cervical cardiac branches
⑦ right recurrent laryngeal n.
⑧ subclavian a.
⑨ cricothyroid
⑩ vagus n. (CN X)

❗ The recurrent laryngeal n., a branch of the vagus n., is closely related to the posterior aspect of the thyroid. Damage to the nerve during surgery can result in paralysis of the ipsilateral vocal cord and intrinsic laryngeal muscles, causing hoarseness.

Fig. 39.22A. From *Atlas of Anatomy, Third Edition*, p. 539.

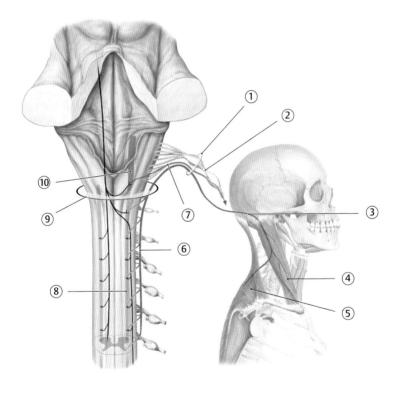

Cranial Nerves: CN XI

①   jugular foramen

②   vagus n. (CN X)

③   accessory n. (CN XI)

④   sternocleidomastoid

⑤   trapezius

⑥   spinal root

⑦   cranial root

⑧   spinal nucleus of accessory n.

⑨   foramen magnum

⑩   nucleus ambiguus

The cranial root of the accessory n. (CN XI) is considered a part of the vagus n. (CN X) that travels with the spinal root for a short distance before splitting off. The cranial root fibers are distributed via the vagus n., while the spinal root fibers continue on as the accessory n.

Fig. 39.23. From *Atlas of Anatomy, Third Edition*, p. 540.

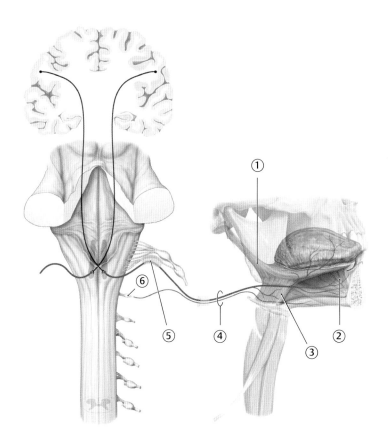

How would a unilateral lesion of the hypoglossal n. (CN XII) present in a patient?

Cranial Nerves: CN XII

① styloglossus

② genioglossus

③ hyoglossus

④ hypoglossal n. (CN XII)

⑤ hypoglossal canal

⑥ C1 spinal n.

⚠ The hypoglossal n. (CN XII) innervates muscles of the tongue. A lesion of the nerve would cause the protruded tongue to deviate to the side of the injury.

Fig. 39.25. From *Atlas of Anatomy, Third Edition*, p. 541.

Motor Innervation of the Face

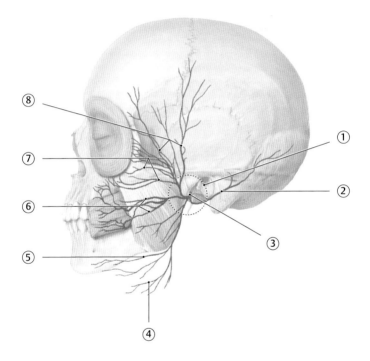

🅿 Which muscles of the face are not innervated by the facial n. (CN VII)?

Motor Innervation of the Face

① parotid plexus

② posterior auricular n.

③ facial n. (CN VII)

④ cervical branch

⑤ marginal mandibular branch

⑥ buccal branches

⑦ zygomatic branches

⑧ temporal branches

⚠ The facial n. innervates all muscles of facial expression. The muscles of mastication, however, are innervated by the mandibular division of the trigeminal n. (CN V₃).

Fig. 40.1A. From *Atlas of Anatomy, Third Edition*, p. 544.

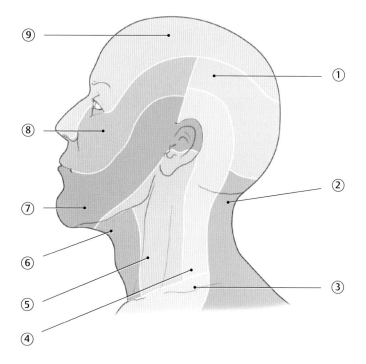

Sensory Innervation of the Head and Neck

① greater occipital n. (C2)

② spinal nn., posterior rami

③ supraclavicular nn.

④ lesser occipital n.

⑤ great auricular n.

⑥ transverse cervical n.

⑦ mandibular division (CN V_3)

⑧ maxillary division (CN V_2)

⑨ ophthalmic division (CN V_1)

Fig. 40.2B. From *Atlas of Anatomy, Third Edition*, p. 545.

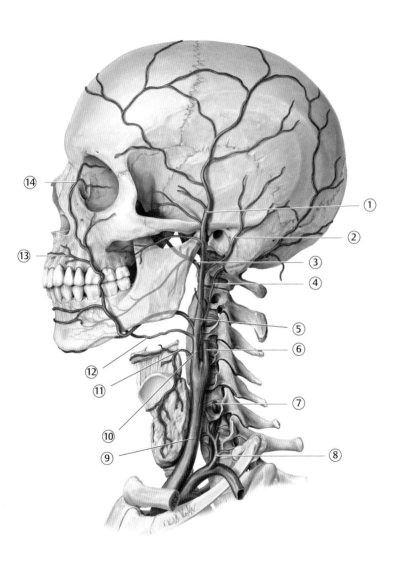

External Carotid Artery

① superficial temporal a.
② posterior auricular a.
③ maxillary a.
④ occipital a.
⑤ facial a.
⑥ internal carotid a.
⑦ vertebral a.
⑧ thyrocervical trunk
⑨ left common carotid a.
⑩ external carotid a.
⑪ superior thyroid a.
⑫ lingual a.
⑬ superior labial a.
⑭ angular a.

Branches of the external carotid artery	
Group	Artery
Anterior	Superior thyroid a.
	Lingual a.
	Facial a.
Medial	Ascending pharyngeal a.
Posterior	Occipital a.
	Posterior auricular a.
Terminal	Maxillary a.
	Superficial temporal a.

Fig. 40.4B. From *Atlas of Anatomy, Third Edition*, p. 547.

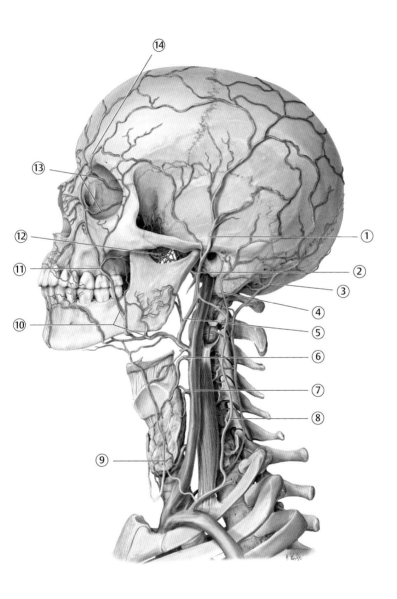

Superficial Veins of the Head and Neck

① superficial temporal v.

② maxillary v.

③ occipital v.

④ posterior auricular v.

⑤ retromandibular v.

⑥ superior thyroid v.

⑦ internal jugular v.

⑧ external jugular v.

⑨ anterior jugular v.

⑩ facial v.

⑪ angular v.

⑫ pterygoid plexus

⑬ superior and inferior ophthalmic vv.

⑭ supraorbital v.

❋ The ophthalmic and deep temporal vv. act as anastomoses between the superficial veins of the face and the dural venous sinuses. Because these veins are valveless, there is a high risk of bacterial dissemination into the cranial cavity from facial infections.

Fig. 40.9B. From *Atlas of Anatomy, Third Edition*, p. 552.

Dural Septa

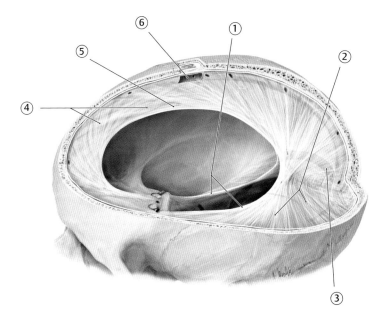

❓ Describe the parts of the brain that are separated by the major dural septa.

Dural Septa

①   tentorial notch

②   tentorium cerebelli

③   transverse sinus

④   falx cerebri

⑤   inferior sagittal sinus

⑥   superior sagittal sinus

! There are three major septa that arise as infoldings of the dura mater: the falx cerebri separates the right and left cerebral hemispheres, the falx cerebelli separates the two cerebellar hemispheres, and the tentorium cerebelli separates the occipital lobe from the cerebellum.

Fig. 40.13. From *Atlas of Anatomy, Third Edition*, p. 554.

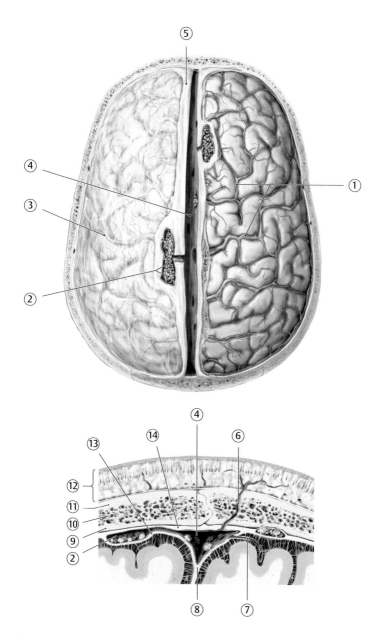

What is the function of the arachnoid granulations?

Superior Sagittal Sinus

① superior cerebral vv.

② arachnoid granulations in lateral lacunae

③ arachnoid mater

④ superior sagittal sinus

⑤ dura mater (cut)

⑥ emissary v.

⑦ bridging v.

⑧ falx cerebri

⑨ inner table

⑩ diploë

⑪ outer table

⑫ scalp

⑬ dura mater, meningeal layer

⑭ dura mater, periosteal layer

📖 Arachnoid granulations are the site of reabsorption of cerebrospinal fluid into the dural venous sinuses.

Fig. 40.12B, Fig. 40.16A. From *Atlas of Anatomy, Third Edition*, pp. 554, 556.

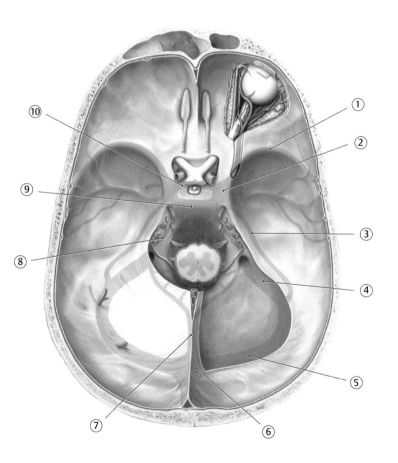

Dural Sinuses in the Cranial Cavity

① sphenoparietal sinus

② cavernous sinus

③ superior petrosal sinus

④ sigmoid sinus

⑤ transverse sinus

⑥ confluence of sinuses

⑦ straight sinus

⑧ inferior petrosal sinus

⑨ posterior intercavernous sinus

⑩ anterior intercavernous sinus

Fig. 40.17. From *Atlas of Anatomy, Third Edition*, p. 556.

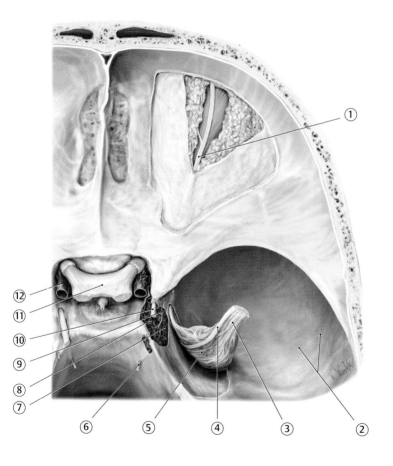

Cavernous Sinus I

① frontal n.
② middle cranial fossa
③ trigeminal n. (CN V) sensory root
④ trigeminal n. (CN V), motor root
⑤ trigeminal ganglion
⑥ abducent n. (CN VI)
⑦ cavernous sinus
⑧ internal carotid a.
⑨ trochlear n. (CN IV)
⑩ oculomotor n. (CN III)
⑪ optic chiasm (optic n., CN II)
⑫ internal carotid a.

Fig. 40.18. From *Atlas of Anatomy, Third Edition*, p. 557.

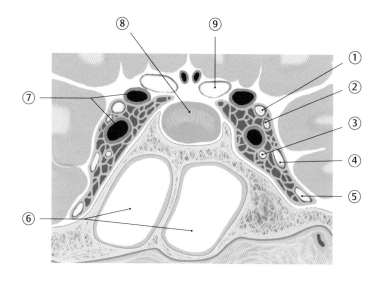

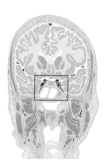

Cavernous Sinus II

1. oculomotor n. (CN III)
2. trochlear n. (CN IV)
3. abducent n. (CN VI)
4. ophthalmic n. (CN V$_1$)
5. maxillary n. (CN V$_2$)
6. sphenoid sinus
7. internal carotid a.
8. hypophysis
9. optic n. (CN II)

With the exception of the optic n., all cranial nerves entering the orbit first pass through the cavernous sinus. The occulomotor and trochlear nn., and the ophthalmic division of the trigeminal n. course along its lateral wall. The abducent n., however, passes through the center of the sinus in close proximity to the internal carotid artery and therefore is the most likely to be affected by an intercavernous aneurysm.

Fig. 40.19. From *Atlas of Anatomy, Third Edition*, p. 557.

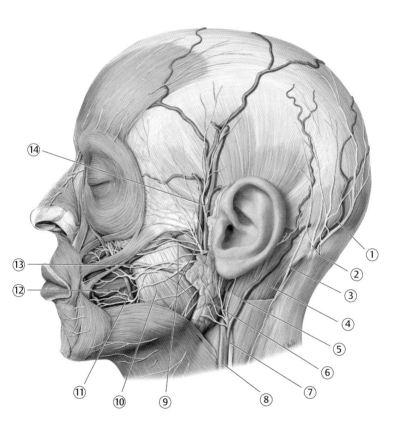

What structure is most at risk during removal of a parotid tumor?

Superficial Neurovasculature of the Head

1. occipital a.
2. greater occipital n. (C2 posterior rami)
3. lesser occipital n. (C2 from cervical plexus)
4. sternocleidomastoid
5. posterior auricular v.
6. parotid gland
7. great auricular n.
8. external jugular v.
9. parotid plexus
10. masseter
11. facial v.
12. buccinator
13. parotid duct
14. auriculotemporal n.

The facial n. (CN VII) passes through and divides within the parotid gland. Its branches are therefore, at high risk of injury during removal of the gland.

Fig. 40.21. From *Atlas of Anatomy, Third Edition*, p. 559.

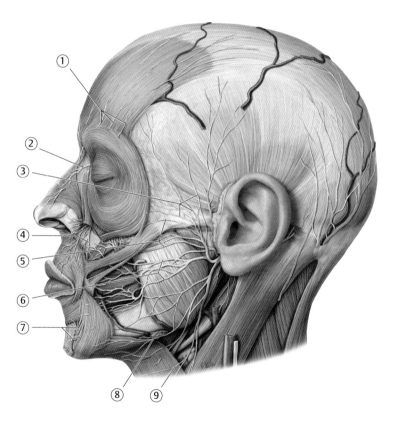

Parotid Region

① supraorbital n (CN V_1)

② infratrochlear n. (CN V_1)

③ temporal branches, parotid plexus (CN VII)

④ infraorbital n. (CN V_2)

⑤ zygomatic branches, parotid plexus (CN VII)

⑥ buccal branches, parotid plexus (CN VII)

⑦ mental n. (CN V_3)

⑧ marginal mandibular branch., parotid plexus (CN VII)

⑨ cervical branch, parotid plexus (CN VII)

Fig. 40.22. From *Atlas of Anatomy, Third Edition*, p. 560.

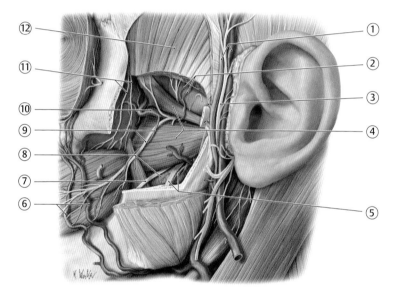

①
②
③
④
⑤
⑥
⑦
⑧
⑨
⑩
⑪
⑫

Infratemporal Fossa: Superficial Layer

① superficial temporal a. and v.
② deep temporal aa.
③ auriculotemporal n. (CN V_3)
④ lateral pterygoid, superior and inferior heads
⑤ inferior alveolar a. and n. (CN V_3)
⑥ facial a. and v.
⑦ lingual n. (CN V_3)
⑧ medial pterygoid, superficial and deep heads
⑨ buccal a. and n. (CN V_3)
⑩ maxillary a.
⑪ superior alveolar nn. (CN V_2)
⑫ temporalis (cut)

Fig. 40.25. From *Atlas of Anatomy, Third Edition*, p. 562.

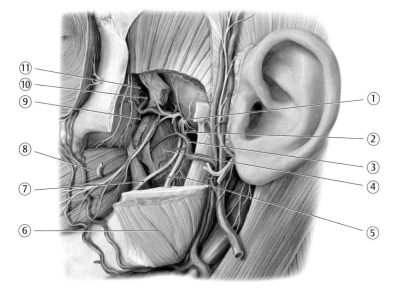

Nerves of the infratemporal fossa are predominantly branches of the mandibular division (CN V$_3$). Through which opening does this nerve exit the base of the skull?

Infratemporal Fossa: Deep Layer

① trigeminal n., mandibular division (CN V$_3$)

② middle meningeal a.

③ maxillary a.

④ medial pterygoid, deep head

⑤ inferior alveolar a. and n. (CN V$_3$)

⑥ masseter

⑦ lingual n. (CN V$_3$)

⑧ buccinator

⑨ posterior superior alveolar a.

⑩ sphenopalatine a.

⑪ infraorbital a.

❗ The mandibular division passes through the foramen ovale of the middle cranial fossa to enter the infratemporal fossa.

Fig. 40.26. From *Atlas of Anatomy, Third Edition*, p. 563.

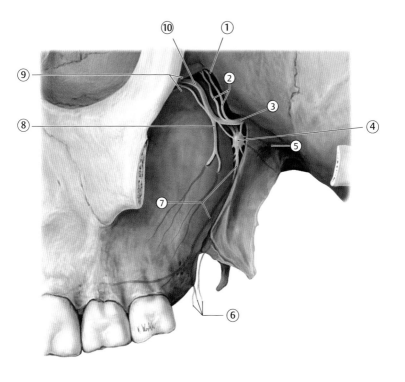

Nerves of the Pterygopalatine Fossa

① pterygomaxillary fissure
② orbital branches from CN V_2
③ maxillary n. (CN V_2)
④ pterygopalatine ganglion
⑤ n. of pterygoid canal
⑥ lesser palatine nn.
⑦ greater palatine n.
⑧ posterior superior alveolar n.
⑨ inferior orbital fissure
⑩ infraorbital n.

✳ The small pyramid-shaped pterygopalatine fossa is a passageway for neurovascular structures (such as the maxillary division of the trigeminal n. and its branches) traveling between the middle cranial fossa and the orbit, nasal cavity, and oral cavity. *Postganglionic sympathetic* fibers from the deep petrosal n. pass uninterrupted through the fossa, whereas *preganglionic parasympathetic* fibers of the greater petrosal n. synapse in the pterygopalatine ganglion.

Fig. 40.29. From *Atlas of Anatomy, Third Edition*, p. 565.

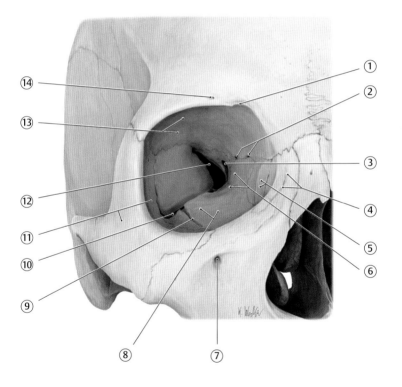

Bones of the Orbit

1. frontal incisure
2. anterior and posterior ethmoidal foramina
3. optic canal
4. maxilla, frontal process
5. lacrimal bone
6. ethmoid bone, orbital plate
7. infraorbital foramen
8. maxilla, orbital surface
9. infraorbital groove
10. inferior orbital fissure
11. zygomatic bone
12. superior orbital fissure
13. frontal bone , orbital surface
14. supraorbital foramen

Fig. 41.1A. From *Atlas of Anatomy, Third Edition*, p. 566.

Coronal Section of the Facial Skeleton

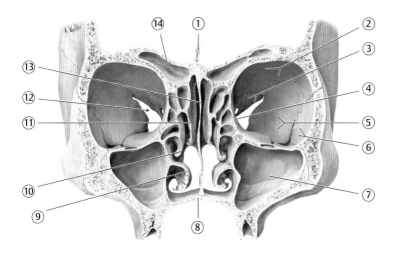

? Which bones of the skull contain paranasal sinuses?

Coronal Section of the Facial Skeleton

1. ethmoid bone, crista galli
2. frontal bone, orbital surface
3. sphenoid bone lesser wing
4. ethmoid bone, orbital plate
5. sphenoid bone, greater wing
6. zygomatic, orbital surface
7. maxillary sinus
8. maxilla, palatine process
9. inferior nasal concha
10. ethmoid bone, middle nasal concha
11. ethmoid bone, superior nasal concha
12. superior orbital fissure
13. ethmoid bone, perpendicular plate
14. frontal sinus

⚠ Paranasal sinuses are found in the frontal, sphenoid, ethmoid, and maxillary bones. All drain into the nasal cavity.

Fig. 41.1D. From *Atlas of Anatomy, Third Edition*, p. 567.

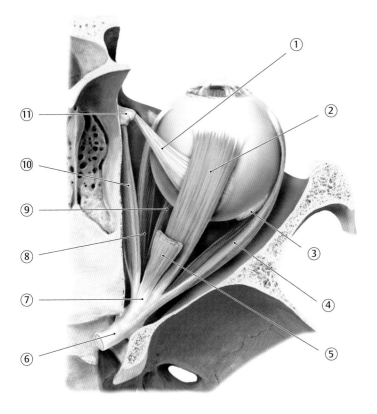

Muscles of the Orbit

① tendon of superior oblique

② superior rectus

③ inferior oblique (insertion)

④ lateral rectus

⑤ levator palpebrae superioris

⑥ optic n. (CN II)

⑦ common tendinous ring

⑧ medial rectus

⑨ inferior rectus

⑩ superior oblique

⑪ trochlea

Muscle	Origin	Insertion	Action*			Innervation
			Vertical axis	Horizontal axis	Anteroposterior axis	
Superior rectus	Common tendinous ring (common annular tendon)	Sclera of the eye	Elevates	Adducts	Rotates medially	Oculomotor n. (CN III), superior branch
Medial rectus			—	Adducts	—	Oculomotor n. (CN III), inferior branch
Inferior rectus			Depresses	Adducts	Rotates laterally	
Lateral rectus			—	Abducts	—	Abducent n. (CN VI)
Superior oblique	Sphenoid bone†		Depresses	Abducts	Rotates medially	Trochlear n. (CN IV)
Inferior oblique	Medial orbital margin		Elevates	Abducts	Rotates laterally	Oculomotor n. (CN III), inferior branch

*Starting from gaze directed anteriorly. †The tendon of the superior oblique passes through a tendinous loop (trochlea) attached to the superomedial orbital margin.

Fig. 41.2B. From *Atlas of Anatomy, Third Edition*, p. 568.

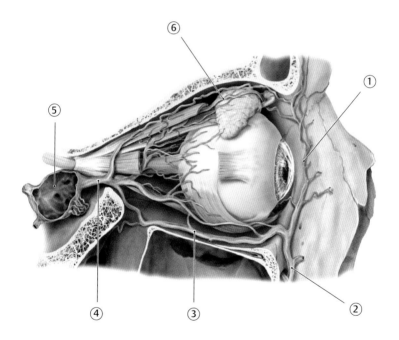

Veins of the Orbit

① angular v.
② facial v.
③ inferior ophthalmic v.
④ ophthalmic v.
⑤ cavernous sinus
⑥ superior ophthalmic v.

Fig. 41.6. From *Atlas of Anatomy, Third Edition*, p. 570.

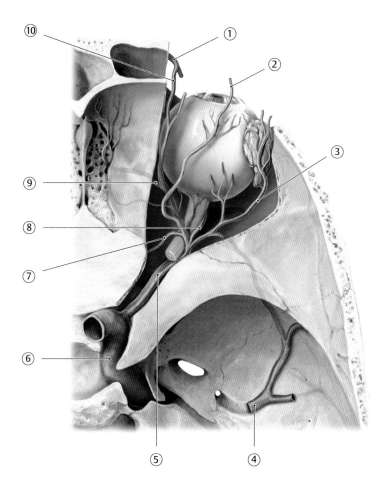

Arteries of the Orbit

- ① dorsal nasal a. (from angular a.)
- ② supraorbital a.
- ③ lacrimal a.
- ④ middle meningeal a.
- ⑤ ophthalmic a.
- ⑥ internal carotid a. in cavernous sinus
- ⑦ posterior ethmoidal a.
- ⑧ central retinal a.
- ⑨ anterior ethmoidal a.
- ⑩ supratrochlear a.

Fig. 41.7. From *Atlas of Anatomy, Third Edition*, p. 570.

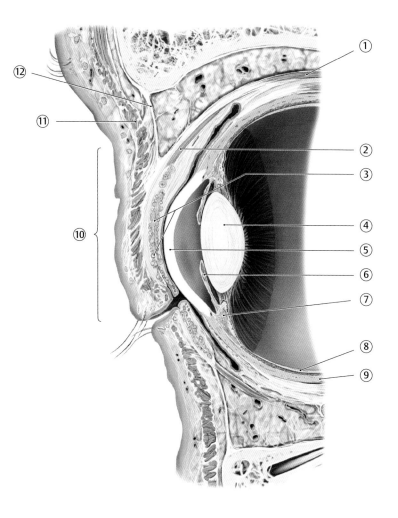

Anterior Orbit and Eyelids

① levator palpebrae superioris
② superior tarsal m.
③ superior tarsus (with tarsal glands)
④ lens
⑤ cornea
⑥ iris
⑦ ciliary body
⑧ retina
⑨ sclera
⑩ upper eyelid
⑪ orbicularis oculi
⑫ orbital septum

Fig. 41.14. From *Atlas of Anatomy, Third Edition*, p. 574.

Structure of the Eyeball

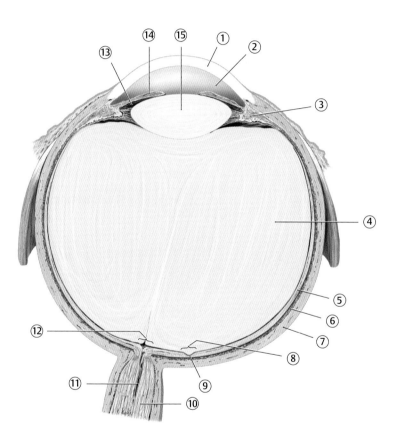

What is glaucoma?

Structure of the Eyeball

① cornea

② anterior chamber

③ ciliary body, ciliary m.

④ vitreous body

⑤ retina

⑥ choroid

⑦ sclera

⑧ macula lutea

⑨ fovea centralis

⑩ optic n. (CN II)

⑪ central retinal a.

⑫ optic disk

! Glaucoma is a condition of increased intraocular pressure caused by a disturbance in the production or drainage of the aqueous humor in the anterior and posterior chambers. The increased pressure can constrict the optic n. where it emerges from the eyeball through the sclera, eventually leading to blindness.

Fig. 41.16. From *Atlas of Anatomy, Third Edition*, p. 576.

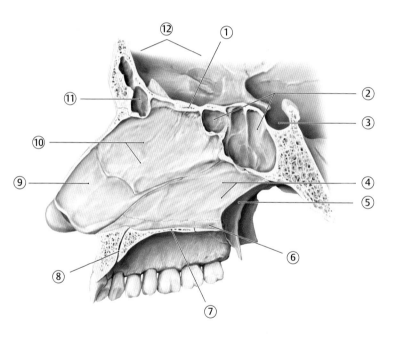

Bones of the Nasal Cavity I: Nasal Septum

①   cribriform plate

②   sphenoid sinus

③   hypophyseal fossa

④   vomer

⑤   choana

⑥   palatine bone, horizontal plate

⑦   maxilla, palatine process

⑧   incisive canal

⑨   septal cartilage

⑩   ethmoid bone, perpendicular plate

⑩   frontal sinus

⑩   anterior cranial fossa

Fig. 42.2A. From *Atlas of Anatomy, Third Edition*, p. 580.

Bones of the Nasal Cavity II: Right Lateral Wall, Concha Removed

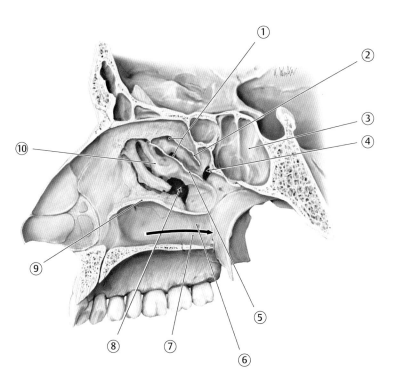

Which of the paranasal sinuses drain into the middle meatus?

Bones of the Nasal Cavity II: Right Lateral Wall, Concha Removed

① orifices of posterior ethmoid sinus

② superior concha (cut)

③ sphenoid sinus

④ sphenopalatine foramen

⑤ middle concha (cut)

⑥ inferior meatus

⑦ palatine bone, perpendicular plate

⑧ maxillary hiatus

⑨ inferior concha (cut)

⑩ ethmoid bulla

⚠ The frontal, maxillary, and anterior and middle ethmoidal paranasal sinuses drain into the middle meatus. The sphenoid sinus drains more superiorly into the sphenoethmoid recess, and the posterior ethmoid sinus drains into the superior meatus. Only the nasolacrimal duct drains to the inferior meatus.

Fig. 42.2C. From *Atlas of Anatomy, Third Edition*, p. 581.

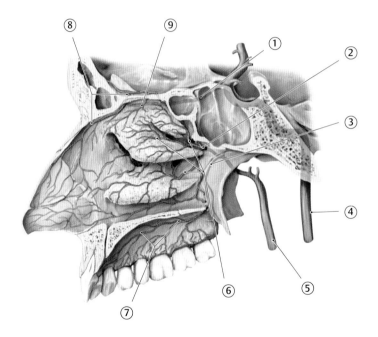

Arteries of the Nasal Cavity

① ophthalmic a.

② sphenopalatine a.

③ descending palatine a.

④ internal carotid a.

⑤ maxillary a.

⑥ lateral posterior nasal aa.

⑦ greater palatine a.

⑧ anterior ethmoid a.

⑨ posterior ethmoid a.

❊ The nasal cavity is a highly vascularized region, supplied by anastomosing branches of the internal carotid a. (ethmoidal branches via the ophthalmic a.) and external carotid a. (sphenopalatine a. via the maxillary a.).

Fig. 42.7B. From *Atlas of Anatomy, Third Edition*, p. 584.

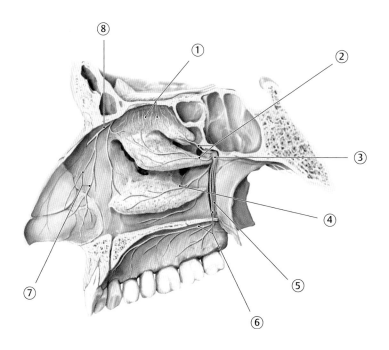

Nerves of the Nasal Cavity

① olfactory fibers (CN I)
② lateral superior posterior nasal branches
③ pterygopalatine ganglion
④ inferior posterior nasal branch
⑤ lesser palatine nn.
⑥ greater palatine n.
⑦ lateral nasal branches
⑧ anterior ethmoidal n. (CN V_1)

Fig. 42.9B. From *Atlas of Anatomy, Third Edition*, p. 585.

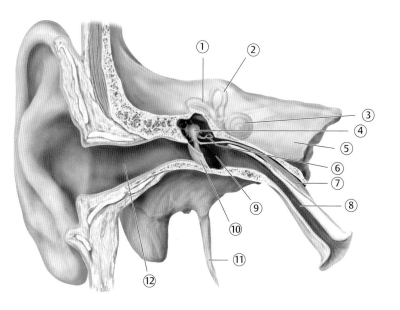

External Ear and Auditory Canal

1. lateral semicircular canal
2. anterior semicircular canal
3. cochlea
4. malleus
5. temporal bone, petrous part
6. stapes
7. tensor tympani
8. pharyngotympanic (auditory) tube
9. tympanic cavity
10. tympanic membrane
11. styloid process
12. external auditory canal

Fig. 43.3. From *Atlas of Anatomy, Third Edition*, p. 588.

Structure of the Auricle

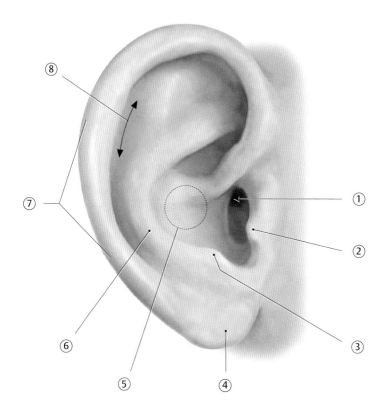

Structure of the Auricle

1. external auditory canal
2. tragus
3. antitragus
4. earlobe
5. concha
6. antihelix
7. helix
8. scaphoid fossa

Fig. 43.5. From *Atlas of Anatomy, Third Edition*, p. 589.

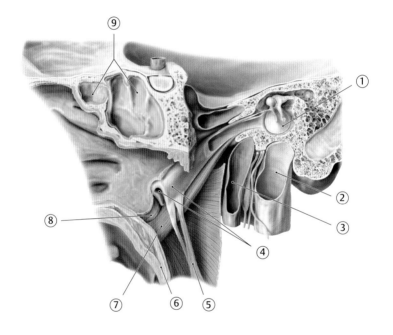

How is pressure in the middle ear equalized by swallowing or yawning?

Tympanic Cavity and Pharyngotympanic Tube

① tympanic membrane
② internal jugular v.
③ internal carotid a.
④ pharyngotympanic tube
⑤ salpingopharyngeus
⑥ uvula
⑦ levator veli palatini
⑧ tensor veli palatini
⑨ sphenoid sinus

▮▮ Muscles of the soft palate, the tensor veli palatini and levator veli palatini, and the salpingopharyngeus muscle function to open the pharyngotympanic tube during swallowing, which relieves pressure in the middle ear.

Fig. 43.9. From *Atlas of Anatomy, Third Edition*, p. 590.

Ossicular Chain in the Tympanic Cavity, Lateral View, Right Ear

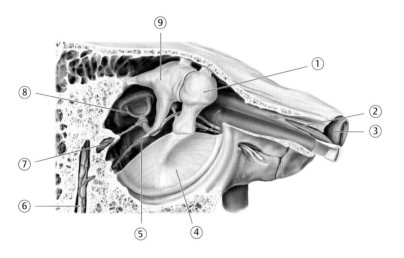

🔲 What is the function of the stapedius and tensor tympani muscles?

Ossicular Chain in the Tympanic Cavity, Lateral View, Right Ear

① malleus
② tensor tympani
③ internal carotid a.
④ tympanic membrane
⑤ chorda tympani
⑥ facial n. (CN VII)
⑦ stapedius m.
⑧ stapes
⑨ incus

⚠ The stapedius and tensor tympani function to reduce sound transmission in the middle ear. Both undergo a reflex contraction in response to loud acoustic stimuli.

Fig. 43.16. From *Atlas of Anatomy, Third Edition*, p. 593.

Auditory Apparatus

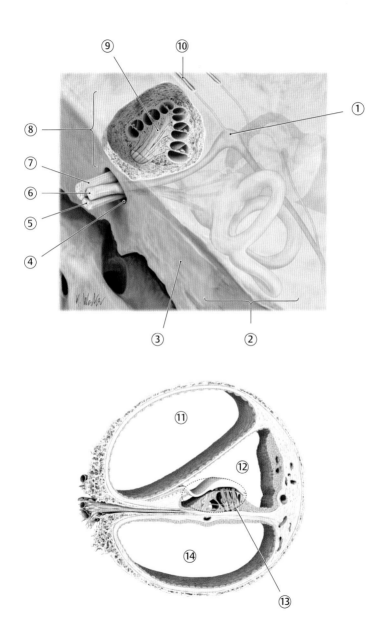

Auditory Apparatus

1. geniculate ganglion
2. semicircular canals
3. temporal bone, petrous part
4. internal acoustic meatus
5. vestibular n. (CN VIII)
6. facial n. (CN VII)
7. cochlear n. (CN VIII)
8. cochlea
9. modiolus
10. greater petrosal n.
11. scala vestibuli
12. cochlear duct
13. organ of Corti
14. scala tympani

Mandible

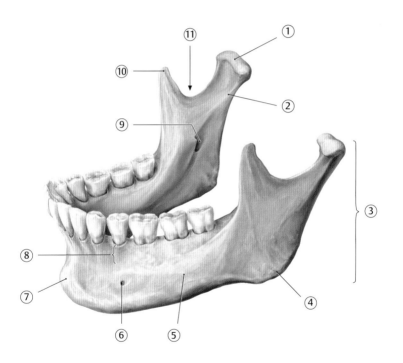

Mandible

1. head (condyle)
2. condylar process
3. ramus
4. angle
5. body
6. mental foramen
7. mental protuberance
8. alveolar process
9. mandibular foramen
10. coronoid process
11. mandibular notch

Fig. 44.2C. From *Atlas of Anatomy, Third Edition*, p. 599.

Suprahyoid Muscles

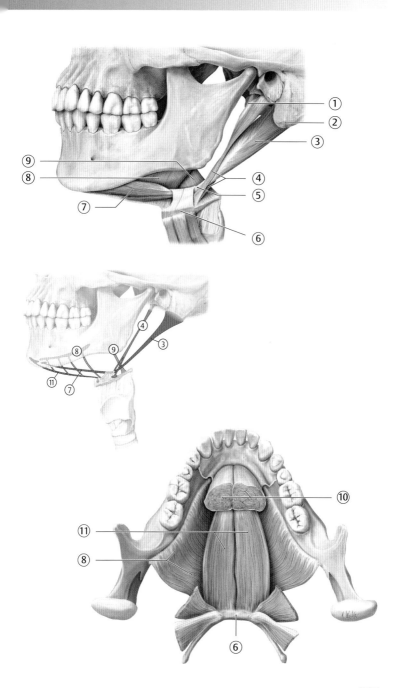

Suprahyoid Muscles

①   styloid process

②   mastoid process

③   digastric, posterior belly

④   stylohyoid

⑤   digastric, intermediate tendon

⑥   hyoid bone

⑦   digastric, anterior belly

⑧   mylohyoid

⑨   hyoglossus

⑩   genioglossus

⑪   geniohyoid

Muscle		Origin	Insertion	Innervation	Action
Digastric	Anterior belly	Mandible (digastric fossa)	Hyoid bone (body)	Mylohyoid n. (from CN V₃)	Elevates hyoid bone (during swallowing), assists in opening mandible
	Posterior belly	Temporal bone (mastoid notch, medial to mastoid process)		Facial n. (CN VII)	
Stylohyoid		Temporal bone (styloid process)			
Mylohyoid		Mandible (mylohyoid line)		Mylohyoid n. (from CN V₃)	Tightens and elevates oral floor, draws hyoid bone forward (during swallowing), assists in opening mandible and moving it side to side (mastication)
Geniohyoid		Mandible (inferior mental spine)		Anterior ramus of C1 via hypoglossal n. (CN XII)	Draws hyoid bone forward (during swallowing), assists in opening mandible
Hyoglossus		Hyoid bone (superior border of greater cornu)	Sides of tongue	Hypoglossal n. (CN XII)	Depresses the tongue

Fig. 44.13A,B,D. From *Atlas of Anatomy, Third Edition*, p. 604.

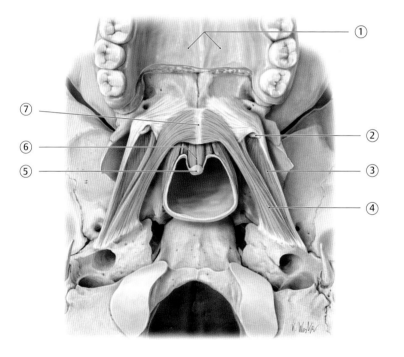

Muscles of the Soft Palate

①   hard palate

②   pterygoid hamulus

③   tensor veli palatini

④   levator veli palatini

⑤   uvula

⑥   musculus uvulae

⑦   palatine aponeurosis

Muscle	Origin	Insertion	Innervation	Action
Tensor veli palatini	Medial pterygoid plate (scaphoid fossa); sphenoid bone (spine); cartilage of pharyngotympanic tube	Palatine aponeurosis	Medial pterygoid n. (CN V_3 via otic ganglion)	Tightens soft palate; opens inlet to pharyngotympanic (auditory) tube (during swallowing, yawning)
Levator veli palatini	Cartilage of pharyngotympanic tube; temporal bone (petrous part)		Vagus n. via pharyngeal plexus	Raises soft palate to horizontal position
Musculus uvulae	Uvula (mucosa)	Palatine aponeurosis; posterior nasal spine		Shortens and raises uvula

Fig. 44.14. From *Atlas of Anatomy, Third Edition*, p. 605.

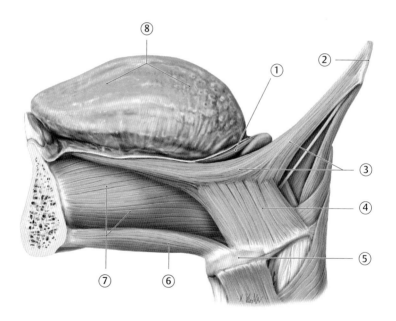

Muscles of the Tongue

① palatoglossus
② styloid process
③ styloglossus
④ hyoglossus
⑤ hyoid bone
⑥ geniohyoid
⑦ genioglossus
⑧ dorsum of tongue

✳ The extrinsic tongue muscles (genioglossus, hyoglossus, palatoglossus, and styloglossus) have bony attachments and move the tongue as a whole. The intrinsic muscles (superior and inferior longitudinal muscles and transverse and vertical muscles) have no bony attachments and merely alter the shape of the tongue.

Fig. 44.19A. From *Atlas of Anatomy, Third Edition*, p. 608.

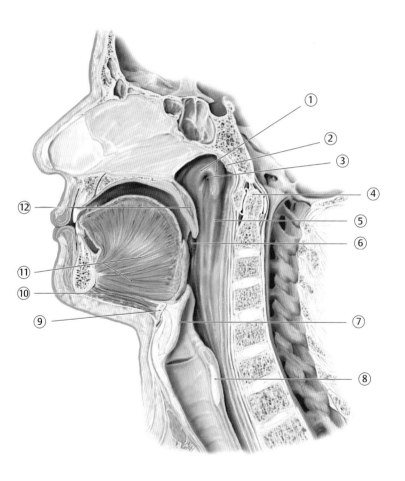

Pharynx and Oral Cavity

① torus tubarius with tubal tonsils
② pharyngeal tonsil
③ pharyngeal orifice of pharyngotympanic tube
④ dens of axis
⑤ salpingopharyngeal fold
⑥ palatine tonsil
⑦ epiglottis
⑧ cricoid cartilage
⑨ hyoid bone
⑩ geniohyoid
⑪ genioglossus
⑫ soft palate

Fig. 44.23B. From *Atlas of Anatomy, Third Edition*, p. 610.

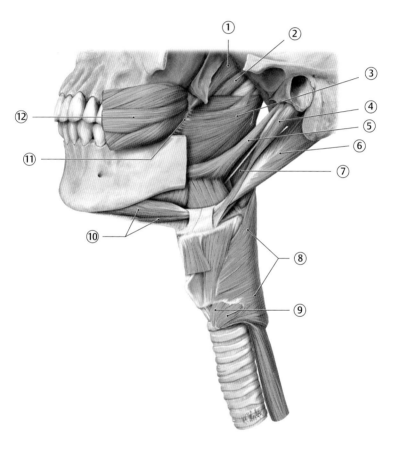

Pharyngeal Muscles I

① tensor veli palatini

② levator veli palatini

③ superior pharyngeal constrictor

④ stylohyoid

⑤ styloglossus

⑥ digastric, posterior belly

⑦ stylopharyngeus

⑧ inferior pharyngeal constrictor

⑨ cricothyroid

⑩ digastric, anterior belly

⑪ pterygomandibular raphe

⑫ buccinator

Fig. 44.28A. From *Atlas of Anatomy, Third Edition*, p. 614.

Pharyngeal Muscles II, Posterior View

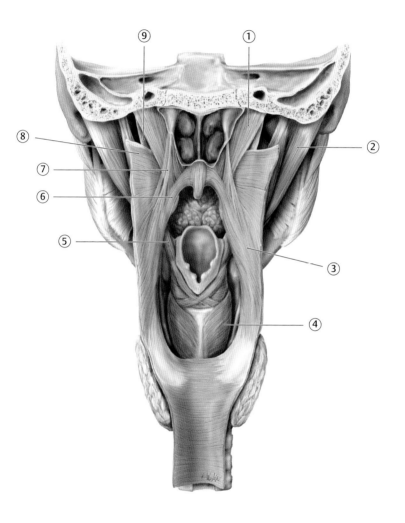

What is the function of the pharyngeal constrictor muscles?

Pharyngeal Muscles II, Posterior View

① levator veli palatini

② digastric, posterior belly

③ middle pharyngeal constrictor

④ posterior cricoarytenoid

⑤ stylopharyngeus

⑥ palatopharyngeus

⑦ salpingopharyngeus

⑧ superior pharyngeal constrictor

⑨ tensor veli palatini

! The superior, middle, and inferior constrictors assist in swallowing by contracting sequentially to move food from the pharynx to the esophagus.

Fig. 44.29C. From *Atlas of Anatomy, Third Edition*, p. 615.

Infrahyoid Muscles

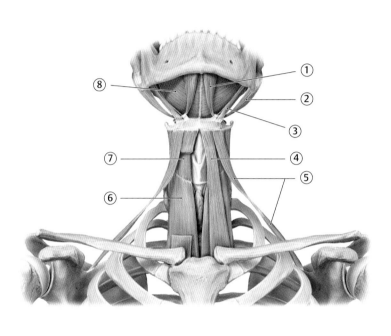

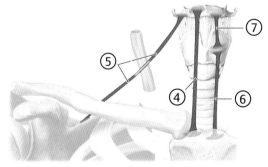

Infrahyoid Muscles

①   digastric, anterior belly

②   digastric, posterior belly

③   stylohyoid

④   sternohyoid

⑤   omohyoid, superior and inferior bellies

⑥   sternothyroid

⑦   thyrohyoid

⑧   mylohyoid

Muscle	Origin	Insertion	Innervation	Action
Omohyoid	Scapula (superior border), inferior belly	Hyoid bone (body), superior belly	Ansa cervicalis (C1–C3) of cervical plexus	Depresses (fixes) hyoid, draws larynx and hyoid down for phonation and terminal phases of swallowing*
Sternohyoid	Manubrium and sternoclavicular joint (posterior surface)			
Sternothyroid	Manubrium (posterior surface)	Thyroid cartilage (oblique line)	Ansa cervicalis (C2–C3) of cervical plexus	
Thyrohyoid	Thyroid cartilage (oblique line)	Hyoid bone (body)	Anterior ramus of C1 via hypoglossal n. (CN XII)	Depresses and fixes hyoid, raises the larynx during swallowing
*The omohyoid also tenses the cervical fascia (via its intermediate tendon).				

Fig. 45.4B, Fig. 45.5C. From *Atlas of Anatomy, Third Edition*, pp. 620, 621.

Cervical Plexus—Sensory Branches

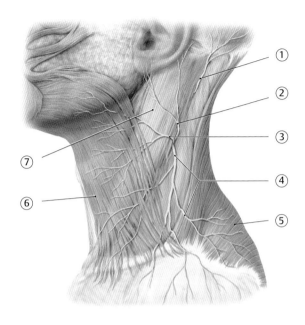

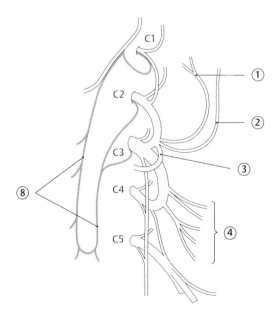

Cervical Plexus—Sensory Branches

① lesser occipital n.

② great auricular n.

③ transverse cervical n.

④ supraclavicular nn.

⑤ trapezius

⑥ platysma

⑦ sternocleidomastoid

⑧ ansa cervicalis

Table 45.8, Fig. 45.14. From *Atlas of Anatomy, Third Edition*, pp. 628, 629.

Cervical Plexus—Motor Branches

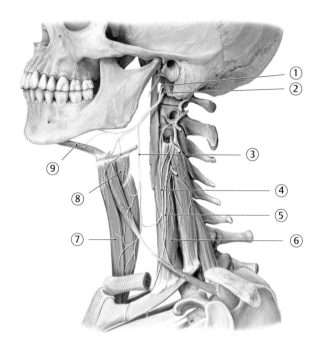

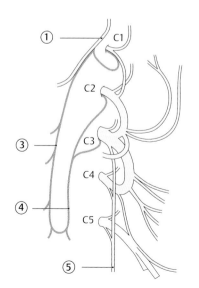

Cervical Plexus—Motor Branches

1. hypoglossal n. (CN XII)
2. C1, anterior ramus
3. superior root of ansa cervicalis
4. inferior root of ansa cervicalis
5. phrenic n.
6. anterior scalene
7. sternohyoid
8. thyrohyoid
9. geniohyoid

Laryngeal Cartilages

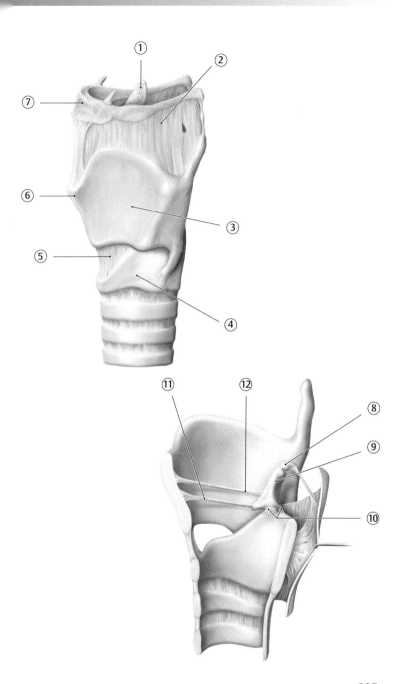

Laryngeal Cartilages

1. epiglottis
2. thyrohyoid membrane
3. thyroid cartilage
4. cricoid cartilage
5. cricothyroid lig.
6. laryngeal prominence
7. hyoid
8. corniculate cartilage
9. arytenoid cartilage
10. cricoarytenoid joint
11. vocal lig.
12. vestibular lig.

Laryngeal Cavity

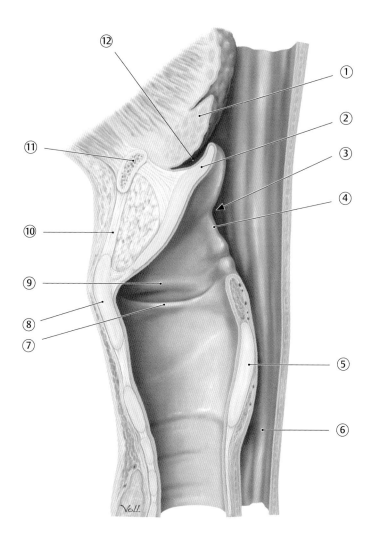

⑦ Which of the intrinsic muscles of the larynx is responsible for abduction of the vocal cords?

Laryngeal Cavity

① lingual tonsil

② epiglottis

③ piriform recess

④ aryepiglottic fold

⑤ cricoid cartilage

⑥ esophagus

⑦ vocal fold

⑧ thyroid cartilage

⑨ vestibular fold

⑩ thyrohyoid lig.

⑪ hyoid

⑫ vallecula

⚠ The posterior cricoarytenoid is the only muscle of the larynx that abducts the vocal cords.

Fig. 45.23B. From *Atlas of Anatomy, Third Edition*, p. 633.

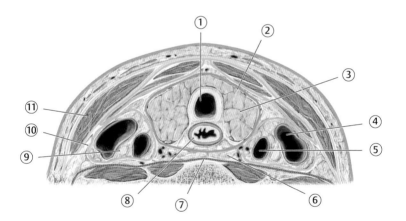

Relations of the Thyroid Gland

① trachea
② pretracheal fascia
③ thyroid gland
④ internal jugular v.
⑤ common carotid a.
⑥ retropharyngeal space
⑦ prevertebral fascia
⑧ esophagus
⑨ vagus n.
⑩ carotid sheath
⑪ sternocleidomastoid

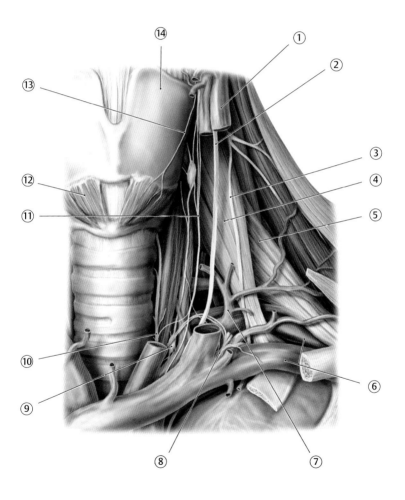

Root of the Neck

1. internal jugular v.
2. vagus n. (CN X)
3. phrenic n.
4. anterior scalene
5. brachial plexus
6. subclavian a. and v.
7. thyrocervical trunk
8. thoracic duct
9. stellate ganglion
10. left recurrent laryngeal n.
11. sympathetic trunk
12. cricothyroid
13. external laryngeal n.
14. thyroid cartilage

Fig. 45.31D. From *Atlas of Anatomy, Third Edition*, p. 639.

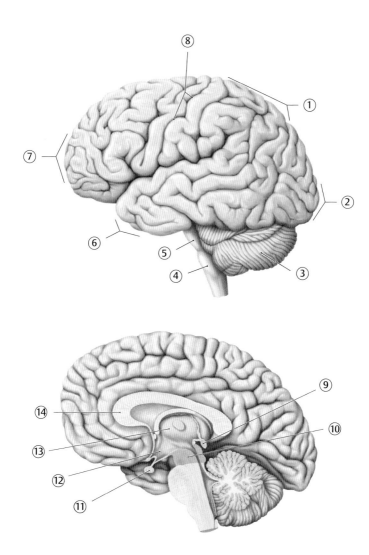

Structure of the Brain

① parietal lobe

② occipital lobe

③ cerebellum

④ medulla oblongata

⑤ pons

⑥ temporal lobe

⑦ frontal lobe

⑧ central sulcus

⑨ pineal gland

⑩ mesencephalon

⑪ hypophysis

⑫ hypothalamus

⑬ thalamus

⑭ corpus callosum

Circulation of Cerebrospinal fluid

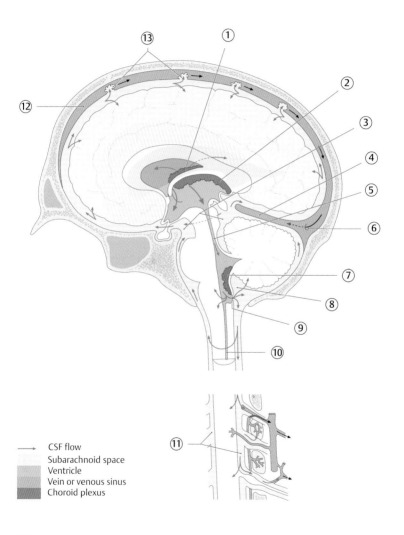

→ CSF flow
Subarachnoid space
Ventricle
Vein or venous sinus
Choroid plexus

? What is hydrocephalus?

Circulation of Cerebrospinal fluid

① choroid plexus (lateral ventricle)

② choroid plexus (3rd ventricle)

③ ambient cistern

④ straight sinus

⑤ cerebral aqueduct

⑥ confluence of sinuses

⑦ choroid plexus (4th ventricle)

⑧ cisterna magna

⑨ median aperture

⑩ central canal of the spinal cord

⑪ subarachnoid space

⑫ superior sagittal sinus

⑬ arachnoid granulations

⚠️ Hydrocephalus is a condition in which there is an excessive accumulation of cerebrospinal fluid (CSF) in the ventricles of the brain. It can result from an obstruction of the flow of CSF within the ventricular system, interference in the reabsorption into the venous system, or rarely, an overproduction of CSF.

Fig. 47.17. From *Atlas of Anatomy, Third Edition*, p. 672.

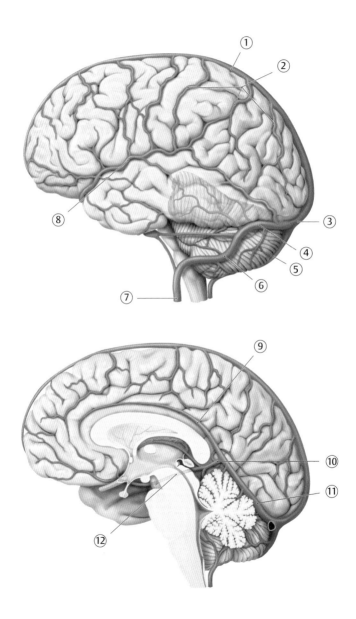

Superficial Cerebral Veins

①   superior sagittal sinus

②   superior cerebral vv.

③   confluence of sinuses

④   transverse sinus

⑤   occipital sinus

⑥   sigmoid sinus

⑦   internal jugular v.

⑧   superficial middle cerebral v.

⑨   inferior sagittal sinus

⑩   great cerebral v.

⑪   straight sinus

⑫   basilar v.

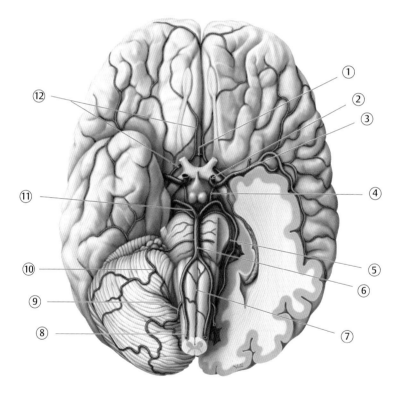

Arteries of the Brain

① anterior communicating a.

② internal carotid a.

③ middle cerebral a.

④ posterior communicating a.

⑤ superior cerebellar a.

⑥ basilar a.

⑦ anterior spinal a.

⑧ vertebral a.

⑨ posterior inferior cerebellar a.

⑩ anterior inferior cerebellar a.

⑪ posterior cerebral a.

⑫ anterior cerebral a.

A stroke is a neurologic deficiency resulting from a cerebral vascular impairment, such as an obstruction of a cerebral artery. Vessels of the circle of Willis can provide collateral circulation to circumvent an obstruction, but anastomoses between vessels may be incomplete or too small to provide adequate circulation.

Fig. 48.6. From *Atlas of Anatomy, Third Edition*, p. 676.

ANS Circuitry

- ⬤ Somatic afferent (sensory)
- ⬤ Somatic efferent (motor)
- ⬤ Sympathetic, preganglionic
- ⬤ Sympathetic, postganglionic
- ⬤ Parasympathetic, preganglionic
- ⬤ Parasympathetic, postganglionic
- ⬤ Visceral afferent (sensory)

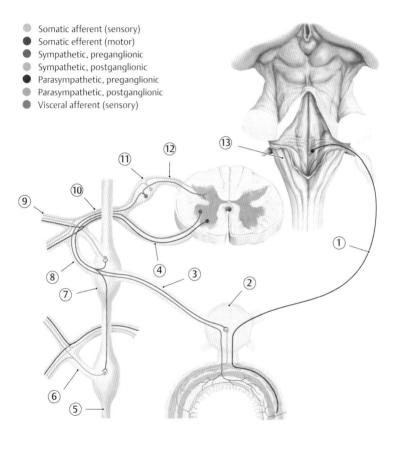

ANS Circuitry

1. vagus n. (preganglionic parasympathetic)
2. prevertebral ganglia
3. splanchnic n.
4. anterior root
5. sympathetic trunk
6. gray ramus communicans
7. paravertebral (sympathetic) ganglion
8. white ramus communicans
9. posterior ramus
10. spinal n. – L2
11. sensory ganglion
12. posterior root
13. brainstem

Fig. 50.3. From *Atlas of Anatomy, Third Edition*, p. 685.